Dances with Spiders

Series: Epistemologies of Healing

General Editors: David Parkin and Elisabeth Hsu: both are at ISCA, Oxford

This series in medical anthropology will publish monographs and collected essays on indigenous (so-called traditional) medical knowledge and practice, alternative and complementary medicine, and ethnobiological studies that relate to health and illness. The emphasis of the series is on the way indigenous epistemologies inform healing, against a background of comparison with other practices, and in recognition of the fluidity between them.

Volume 1
Conjuring Hope: Magic and Healing in Contemporary Russia
Galina Lindquist

Volume 2
Precious Pills: Medicine and Social Change among Tibetan Refugees in India
Audrey Prost

Volume 3
Working with Spirit: Experiencing Izangoma Healing in Contemporary South Africa
Jo Thobeka Wreford

Volume 4
Dances with Spiders: Crisis, Celebrity and Celebration in Southern Italy
Karen Lüdtke

Dances with Spiders

Crisis, Celebrity and Celebration in Southern Italy

Karen Lüdtke

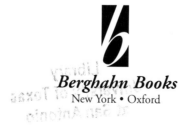

Berghahn Books
New York • Oxford

First published in 2009 by

Berghahn Books

www.berghahnbooks.com

©2009 Karen Lüdtke

Library of Congress Cataloging-in-Publication Data
Ludtke, Karen.
 Dances with spiders : crisis, celebrity and celebration in southern
italy / Karen Ludtke.
  p. cm. -- (Epistemologies of healing ; 4)
 Includes bibliographical references and index.
 ISBN 978-1-84545-445-6 (hardback : alk. paper)
 1. Tarantella--Italy--Salentina Peninsula. 2. Tarantism--Italy--
Salentina Peninsula. 3. Medical anthropology--Italy--Salentina
Peninsula. 4. Salentina Peninsula (Italy)--Social life and customs. 5.
Salentina Peninsula (Italy)--Folklore. I. Title.

GV1796.T32L84 2008
306.4'6109457--dc22
                          2008031377

British Library Cataloguing in Publication Data
A catalogue record for this book is available from the British Library
Printed in the United States on acid-free paper

ISBN 978-1-84545-445-6 hardback

Ad un'amica

The belief in the fluid materiality of the soul
is indispensable to the actor's craft ...
to know that a passion is material ...
confers a mastery upon the actor
which makes him equal to a true healer.

Antonin Artaud 1958: 135

Contents

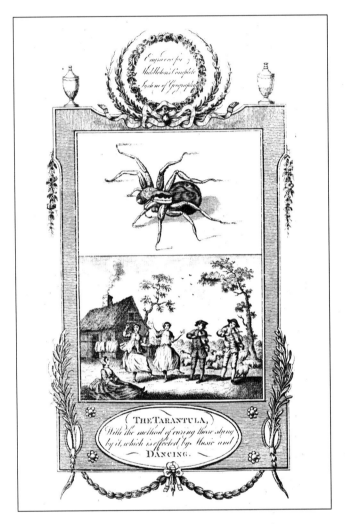

Fig. 0.1 'The tarantula with the method of curing those stung by it, which is effected by music and dancing' (*Middleton's Complete System of Geography*, 18th century) (source: Wellcome Library, London).

List of Illustrations

Acknowledgements

This book has come into existence with the help and inspiration of many who have shared their thoughts and experiences with me over the past ten years.

In the Salento, my gratitude extends to each and every one who has contributed to this study. The words and insights of many make up these pages. The support and kindness of many others, although intangible, lie at the foundation of this book. Giuseppe Leccese first told me about the tarantate and with Marta Visca and Enrico Trevisan accompanied me on my initial visit to the Salento. Ada Metafune and Biagio Panico of the Associazione Novaracne provided a first point of contact and have generously shared their experience ever since. Giorgio Di Lecce and his group Arakne Mediterranea introduced me to the pizzica, welcoming me to their rehearsals, performances and tours.

Giuseppe Memmi, Umberto Panico and Luigi Toma provided important points of reference, as did Roberto Raheli, Edoardo Winspeare, Fabio Tolledi, Sergio Torsello and Daniele Durante.

Luigi Chiriatti took me to St Paul's festival in Galatina in 1997 when everything was new to me. Piero Fumarola, Luigi Santoro, Gianfranco Salvatore, Maurizio Agamennone, Eugenio Imbriani and Gino Di Mitri provided important academic support at various points of my research. Maurizio Nocera showed me 'his' Salento. Fernando Bevilacqua was always ready to share his view, his experiences and a joke. Mariantonietta Colluto and Cosimo Spagnolo introduced me to Evelina and her family, who welcomed me to their home. Vittorio Marras and Bengasi Fai gave me the chance to speak to Francesco Greco, Paolo Zacchino and Luigi Stifani. Rocco Martella contacted me prior to my arrival in the Salento and liberally shared his time and experience to introduce me to people and places he knew. Tonino Asciano spent hours conveying his knowledge about the tambourine's world. Tanya Pagliara trusted me with her experiences. Rita Cappello generously invited me to attend her sessions and courses in the music and art therapy method, 'La globalità dei linguaggi'. Marta Porcino shared many moments of dancing and helped clarify doubts in the final phases of writing.

In England, David Parkin provided me with his guidance, clarity and sensitivity to persevere with this project, offering his help even when I was no longer officially 'under his wing'. Gina Burrows's warmth and friendship have been a constant source of sustenance at the Institute of Social and Cultural Anthropology in Oxford. Murray Last and Hélène La Rue gave important feedback on an earlier draft. Elisabeth Hsu provided helpful comments along the way and her encouragement has always been in the back of my mind. Peregrine Horden has read and saved chapters of the manuscript, stored boxes of fieldwork data in his attic and offered his advice and reassuring sense of humour at crucial points over the years. I also owe the title of this book to him. Hélène Neveu Kringelbach – together with Jonathan Skinner, who first suggested I send a proposal to Berghahn – invited me to participate in the 2004 European Association of Social Anthropologists' panel 'Meaning in Motion: Advancing the Anthropology of Dance'. Jen Cottrill's assistance at Berghahn provided priceless inspiration in the early phases of work on the manuscript, as did the support of Marion Berghahn, Mark Stanton and everyone else at Berghahn in the subsequent stages. Susanne Wessendorf's friendship and feedback spurred on my motivation and reflections, thanks to long discussions about fieldwork in the Salento, even at summer highs in front of the fan, and her diligence in commenting on the manuscript. Marina Roseman's in-depth comments have been fundamental in weaving this study into the broader webs of anthropological studies on music and dance.

Elsewhere, in wind-still moments, Vincenzo Santiglio showed me how to make mind maps. Roberta Greco and Carlo Licci helped reconnect fractured relations. Alessandro De Donno gave untiring logistical aid. Salvatore Manco helped clear dusty spider webs. Paolo de Lorenzo brought out the funny side of things. Linda Safran generously commented on the first draft and final proofs of this book and her friendship, advice and extensive knowledge of the Salento have given me vital boosts of inspiration over the years. Damian Walter liberally shared his thoughts on an earlier draft, as well as valuable references to related publications. Frank Welte inspired me with his knowledge and awareness of therapeutic contexts among the Moroccan Gnawa, and in Germany. Gisela Schmeer told me about her visits to Galatina in the 1970s, enriching my research with her material and insights. Stefano Boni, Mary Ciuffitelli, Jason Dent, James Greer, Luisa Del Giudice, Flavia Laviosa, Michael Palmer and Dorothy Zinn commented on earlier drafts or parts of these, providing precious insights. Dorothy Zinn's English translation of De Martino's book, *The Land of Remorse,* with its valuable footnotes, has been a key point of reference.

Outside the university world, I have treasured the knowledge and experience of Maria Viola Refolo, encouraging me to keep looking. Marcella D'Elia helped me stay where I was and persevere. Jole Lezzi and Mariantonietta Rizzello shared their insights and ideas. Maria Teresa Giampaolo has been a flatmate and friend from the very beginning. Gianni Cacciatore has always been up for a break to swim in the sea. Susanne Etti provided a home for me in Oxford on numerous occasions, read through earlier chapters and shared her enthusiasm and the Salentine world with me. Isha Rubini cheered me on with her passion for existence. Regina Schneider has always highlighted the sunny side and yet another perspective. Kam Raval's friendship has been a point of consistency throughout many changes.

I am indebted to various individuals and institutions for permission to publish their material here. Portions of this book have appeared in my contributions to *Music as Medicine* (Horden 2000), *Performing Ecstasies* (Del Giudice and van Deusen 2005) and *Melissi* (Lüdtke 2005b). Finally, the first part of this research was funded by the Marie Curie Fellowship Scheme of the European Commission and by the Economic and Social Research Council in Britain. The writing up was initially made possible by postdoctoral grants from the Arts and Humanities Research Board and the British Academy. I thank these institutions warmly.

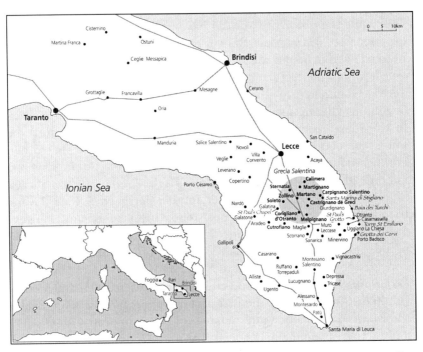

Fig. 0.2 The Salentine peninsula and the region of Apulia (map: Nicki Averill).

Preface

A tiny, elderly woman, enveloped in black, leans against a stone pillar of the gateway leading to her home. Her body is tilted slightly, poised weightlessly against a wall twice her size, one knee bent in adjustment, toes touching, side by side. Her shoulder acts as a pivot, supported by one hand extended across her chest, balancing her dainty shape against the whitewashed bricks. Lost in her gaze, piercing and blue underneath a black headscarf taming strands of beige-white hair, she watches silently.

I look up to check for traffic from behind before turning onto the main road, and find this image framed in my rear mirror. I want to pull out my camera to fix this picture in a permanent frame, but something stops me. Instead, I scan it in my mind and turn to wave, but the scene remains immobile. Her eyes no longer reach this far. Yet they seem to see me departing, simultaneously with many others whom she has accompanied to this gate in farewell, collapsing decades of her life in a single gaze.

She doesn't know if I'll return. I don't know if I'll still find her here again. Over a period of four years (1998–2002), she has promised to come and visit me in England on condition that I leave her a good road map. She has also repeatedly offered to find me a husband in her hometown so I could settle down there. When I return to visit in August 2005, her offer still stands and she extends it to the female friend accompanying me. Her incessant jokes and sunny presence give no hint of the equally strong crises that have marked her life: the sudden fainting spells; the terrorised screams; the shaking that takes over her petite but potent body; the rigidity that leaves her muscles seemingly dead and alive at once.

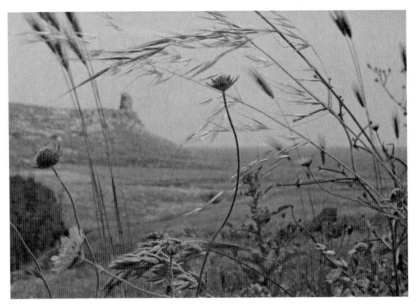

Fig. 0.3 Torre St Emiliano near Porto Badisco on the Adriatic coast, May 2004 (photo: Regina Schneider).

Introduction:
Tarantula Territory

> If we do not honour our past
> we lose our future.
> If we destroy our roots,
> we cannot grow.
>
> Friedensreich Hundertwasser[1]

The Salentine peninsula is an arid, rocky, olive-tree terrain exposed to two main winds and seas. The Tramontana brings cool air across the mountain ranges of northern Italy, blowing the waves of the Ionian Sea onto the sandy shores of the western coast. On the other side, the Scirocco drives desert air from North Africa onto the largely rugged and steep cliffs of the eastern Adriatic coast. Throughout history, these winds and waves have made this far limb of Italian soil into a cultural crossroads at the heart of the Mediterranean, bringing crusaders, invaders, travellers and pilgrims in bygone times, and an influx of refugees and tourists in recent years. It is here, in the heel of Italy's boot, at the southernmost tip of Apulia, that the European black widow, the feared tarantula, reigned in real and mythic terms.

For centuries, the healing cult of tarantism (or tarantolism) was the only cure for those 'bitten' or 'possessed' by the tarantula spider.[2] Its victims had to dance for days on end to the *pizzica* (the Apulian tarantella).[3] Only in this way, it was said, could the spider's poison be expelled and – often temporary – relief be assured. In the post-war period, pesticides were said to have largely eradicated the tarantula from Salentine terrain, and with it, popular belief explains, the tradition of tarantism and its protagonists, the *tarantate* (or *tarantolate*).[4] Subsequent research, bringing socio-economic factors into relief, has inevitably questioned this popular rationalization.

1

Officially, but not quite in practice, tarantism became nothing but a memory, shamefully dismissed or happily relegated to a distant past. However, in the 1990s, the pizzica resurfaced, turning into a local craze mesmerizing masses of dance and music enthusiasts. Reinvented and revitalized, this music has come to attract crowds and sponsors, fabricating and marketing a unique sense of regional identity on the basis of its captivating rhythms and powerful mythic origins.[5]

This book explores how and why the pizzica has boomed in the Salento, creating repercussions on a national and international level. It does so by enquiring whether this current popularity has anything to do with the historical ritual of tarantism, other than as a source of rhetorical legitimation for contemporary forms of the tarantula's music and dance.[6] It asks, more specifically, whether the notion of recovering well-being – in the sense of vitality, presence and choice motivating daily life despite perceived physical or other imperfections – is still of any relevance. A clear picture emerges of the potential of music and dance both to further conflict and to promote well-being, with respect to acute questions of identity in an increasingly globalized world. While conflicts – based on such differences as gender, age, regional origins or musical execution – may be musically played out against each other, experiences in which 'music takes over' may provide a way of sensing and making sense of everyday life beyond such clashing views. In the Salento, a vital shift appears: from the confrontation of life crises to the vibrant promotion and celebration of a local sense of celebrity and identity.[7]

Salentine Tarantulas: Spider Dances and Discourses

The European black widow, alias tarantula, is said to take its name from the Apulian port of Taranto, perched on the convex bend of the Ionian Sea where the heel and arch of Italy's boot meet (Naselli 1951). There is some debate about which spider type was actually associated with the spider's cult, with the *Latrodectus tredecim guttatus* and *Lycosa tarantula* being prime candidates (Lewis 1991).[8] However, unlike its South American counterparts and horror-movie favourites, the so-called Italian tarantula or European black widow

(*Latrodectus tredecim guttatus*) is a petite three centimetres in length and bald, so to speak (Katner 1956). Yet its bite may cause dramatic general symptoms, including severe muscle cramps and convulsions.[9] The region of Apulia, and much of southern Italy, made up its natural habitat. Importantly, however, most cases of tarantism never featured an actual spider bite. No real spider was involved. This is where myth, mystery and symbolism make their powerful entry on stage, a fact that has intrigued thinkers for centuries.

Publications on tarantism, from earliest fourteenth-century manuscripts to twenty-first-century research, have focused primarily on musical, medical, psychological and socio-religious interpretations (Kircher 1641; Baglivi 1696; Hecker 1865; De Raho 1908; Giordano 1957; De Martino 1961a). Some work has drawn on medical anthropology (Lanternari 1995, 2000) or theatre and dance studies (Santoro 1982, 1987; Almiento 1990; Schott-Billmann 1994; Di Lecce 1998). Recent documents on tarantism and its music (Di Lecce 1994; Chiriatti 1995; Chiriatti et al. 2007; Basile 2000; Carignani 2004; Nocera 2005; Agamennone 2005; Romanazzi 2006; Attanasi 2007; Montinaro 2007) and the current musical scene in the Salento (De Giorgi 1999, 2002, 2004, 2005; Nacci 2001, 2004; Lamanna 2002; Santoro and Torsello 2002; Durante 2005; Thayer 2005; Imbriani and Fumarola 2007) provide ethnographic data in Italian and some valuable theoretical insights. The tarantula has also inspired the creativity of various fiction writers (Di Ciaula 2001; Schmeer 2001, Bandini 2006, Marino 2007). Complementary studies on rituals in European and Mediterranean contexts present important comparative material (Boissevain 1992; Ferrari de Nigris 1997; Tak 2000; Del Giudice and van Deusen 2005). Meanwhile, anthropological research on rituals, trance and spirit possession has made reference to tarantism in regard to theoretical discussions on healing and altered states of consciousness (Lewis 1971; Rouget 1986; Lapassade 1994, 1996a, b, 1997, 2001).

This study seeks to develop the existing literature on the basis of fresh data regarding the personal experiences of past and present participants in the tarantula's music and dance, by asking whether the tarantula still 'bites to heal' and what this may reveal about performance and well-being more generally. Since 1953, Evelina has been bitten twice. Every May and June, ever since, she has succumbed to the crises the tarantula evokes: fainting spells, nausea, stomach pains. She is one of the few tarantate who remain in the Salento. Now in her eighties, her story is that of a woman transfixed by taboos. Her life reveals history bodily inscribed, with a complex cultural code channelling her personal anguish. Her story is reminiscent of many others, mainly women, who were struck by traumatic events, harsh living conditions, socially and sexually repressive roles or unspoken judgements, who exploded emotionally, venting their anger and desires in ritualized form, so as to (often temporarily) reinstate a sense of integrity, wholeness, soundness, in the face of everyday life.

By the turn of the millennium, the spider was officially listed as exterminated, eradicated from the land, barring a few exceptions. Evelina is one. Her world is light years away from the current show business that has brought the tarantula's music and dance to fame. Local politicians mingle with pop stars on stage and tourism promotions feed off the eight-legged creature. Once the spider tormented the inhabitants of this region; now it symbolizes sultry summer nights of entertainment and distraction. What is more, nationally and internationally renowned musicians (Joe Zawinul, Noa, Stewart Copeland and others) have been invited to play and take the tarantula on tour. All this has come to make up the so-called world of neo-tarantism.[10]

The Salento makes fertile terrain for exploring the tarantula's music and dance in past and present contexts. Tarantism is extremely well documented historically, as the earliest written references to this phenomenon date back to the fourteenth century (Mina 2000). Similar traditions existed in Sardinia (Gallini 1967), Calabria (Lombardi Satriani 1951), Campania (Rossi 1991) and other regions of Italy (Pitré 1894; Zanetti 1978), as well as Spain (Cid 1787; Doménech y Amaya 1792; Schneider 1948; León Sanz 2000, 2008), but literary evidence of these is comparatively limited. Moreover, cases of tarantism have persisted, in transmuted forms, into the twenty-first century. Although today this phenomenon has largely died out, rare cases were observed until the 1990s, despite modern psychiatric and pharmaceutical alternatives (Di Lecce 1994; Chiriatti 1995; Nocera 2005). What is more, with the turn from the twentieth to the twenty-first century, tarantism has been recast as neo-tarantism. This creates a comparative advantage for looking at the tarantula's music and dance in a single geographical context, both when securely anchored within a strong cultural belief system and when recomposed and reimposed within a new temporal and socio-economic context.

Tarantism is, moreover, a key theme in Italian anthropology, thanks to historian of religion Ernesto De Martino's (1961a) classic study on this topic, *La terra del rimorso*.[11] This major point of reference in research on the tarantula's cult straddles the two main strands of anthropological studies in Italy: folklore studies considering 'folklore' as a response to the historical experience of oppression and as a possible basis of subaltern cultures such as those of the tarantate (De Martino 1960; Gramsci 1985); and cultural anthropology, concerned with the 'value orientations' of individuals living in changing social and economic contexts (Tentori 1976; Tullio-Altan 1976). These emphases much resemble Anglo-American research in the Mediterranean (Saunders 1984; Herzfeld 1987; Driessen 2002) with its consideration of the honour and shame complex (Davis 1969; Peristiany 1965; Schneider and Schneider 1971; Goddard 1987; Giordano 2002), family structures (Banfield 1958; Silverman 1968; Ginsborg 1990), and clientelism and patronage (Filipucci 1996; Gribaudi 1996). Most importantly, the so-called 'Southern Question', probing attempts to explain underdevelopment, as well as sociocultural and economic gaps between Italy's north and its southern regions, or Mezzogiorno, has dominated anthropological studies in recent years, providing a significant contextualization for past and present manifestations of the tarantula's cult (Giordano 1992; Schneider 1998).[12]

In the Salento, the pizzica is generally, simplistically, seen to characterize the traditional music and dance scene, thereby pushing a large repertory of music, including work, love and funeral songs, into the background.[13] Moreover, it is commonly, if reductively and erroneously according to some, divided into three types: the *pizzica tarantata*, *pizzica de core* and *pizzica scherma* (Di Lecce 2001b).[14] All are performed in a circle of participants (both musicians and onlookers), known as *ronda* [see Fig. 9.3], and can be linked by broad similarities in rhythm and musical execution, but distinguished by dance steps, rhythmic subtleties and diverging intentions.[15] The pizzica tarantata was the healing dance of the tarantate performed in a ritual context with the explicit aim of bringing about a greater state of well-being. The pizzica pizzica, pizzica de core or *pizzica di cuore* (literally, 'pizzica of the heart') is danced on social occasions to have fun and to seduce, while the pizzica scherma (literally, fencing pizzica), or simply *scherma*, as many in the know insist, is a fighting dance executed almost exclusively by men.

Controversies regarding terms and neologisms immediately come into the spotlight. Dance ethnologist Giuseppe Gala warns that the term pizzica de core, for instance, is a recent invention: in the past, dances for entertainment were simply known as pizzica pizzica or tarantella.[16] Similarly, the pizzica scherma is often, apparently falsely, considered to be a synonym of the *danza delle spade* (sword dance) or *danza dei coltelli* (knife dance).[17] More recently, the catchphrase *pizzica e taranta* has become common currency with the term 'taranta' signifying not only the spider but also Salentine music and dance more generally. This points to a collapsing of these components in linguistic terms, indicative of the multiple and fluctuating meanings characterizing this performance context.[18] In this study, I adopt the term pizzica pizzica to denote the courtship dance, whereas I use the notion of pizzica in the sense of a music and dance genre (including various types of *pizziche*) holding a key position in the repertory of the tarantula's music and dance, comprising all musical and choreographic events, past and present, orbiting around the spider's image.

Despite the vast quantity of documents on tarantism, limited information is available on the origins of the pizzica, its links to tarantism and its relationship to the southern Italian tarantella more generally (Bragaglia 1949, 1950; Galanti 1950; Costa and Costa 1999; De Giorgi 2002: 53–59). David Gentilcore writes that in the seventeenth century 'the style of dance known as tarantella became widespread throughout the south of Italy' (2000: 265). Generally, however, the ritual form of the tarantella is seen to have come first. The ritual dances of tarantism, which we could call "liturgical", clearly lay behind this "profane" tarantella. In the mid-eighteenth century "to dance like a tarantata" [*ballare a tarantata*] meant to dance the tarantella'[19] (Gentilcore 2000: 265).

Carmelina Naselli (1951) comes to similar conclusions following her investigation into the etymology of the term tarantella. She cites Giorgio Baglivi to explain that one specific tune used during tarantism rituals in the seventeenth century was seen as particularly efficacious and consequently named tarantella, perhaps because its fast rhythm recalled the speed and mobility with which the tarantula spider could move. Yet others asserted that the spider itself moved rhythmically when a tarantella was played [see Fig. 2.1]. Others link tarantism to the tarantella, because the symptoms treated involved an irresistible urge to dance (De Raho 1908: 3). At the same time, dancing the tarantella was also compared to the convulsions of those bitten by the tarantula.[20] Whatever its precise origins the tarantella has evolved into diverse regional styles (Neapolitan, Calabrian and Sicilian, to name just a few) and the Apulian form is generally known as pizzica or pizzica pizzica. Etymological links to the verb *pizzicare*, meaning to 'bite', 'pinch' or 'sting', further evoke the tarantula's presence.

The scherma, meanwhile, is said to derive from prison settings, where dance was a way of settling disputes that could not be voiced otherwise (Monaco 2006). Antonio Gramsci's (1965) observations on these dances are popularly quoted.[21] For those in the know, steps and gestures embody hidden codes. Festive occasions, such as the festival of San Rocco, where the Rom populations of Apulia (earning their living from selling livestock and known for their expertise in dancing) met Salentine farmers (who brought their tambourines and music to pass time and celebrate), are thought to have kept this dance alive (Di Lecce 1992; Melchioni 1999; Tarantino 2001; Chiriatti and Miscuglio 2004; Monaco 2006; Inguscio 2007).

Although classifications of the pizzica are varied and contested, the pizzica pizzica, scherma and pizzica tarantata may be clearly distinguished, despite possibilities of personal variation and change in each new enactment, on the basis of key features seen to characterize each of these dances.[22] The pizzica pizzica marks celebrations and is mostly danced by a man and a woman, although two women (and less frequently two men) may also dance together [see Fig. 9.1]. In the classic match, the woman dances in small skips and pirouettes. She lures and coaxes, escaping her partner while flirting and inviting him to follow with graceful, seductive gestures of her hands, often waving a handkerchief. The man moves more boldly, following his partner, arms seeking to delimit the space around her in a territorial manner, knees slightly bent, assertive and yet almost in submission (Negro and Sergio 2000).

The scherma, in contrast, is used to settle conflicts, frequently over women, to clarify who is the strongest, who has the last say [see

Fig. 9.2]. Two dancers take over the circle centre. Right hands gripped in a tight fist, they turn around the axis of this fulcrum, let go and face each other. Index and middle fingers imitate knives, cutting through the air in rotating motions. The aim is to strike the adversary with force and virility. Tensions run high and electricity moves in the circle, creating sparks with every successful hit. Previously this dance was performed exclusively by men and – as many like to tell and others contest – with actual knives.[23]

Finally, the tarantate danced the pizzica tarantata in spider-driven rituals. Despite vast variations in ritual practices, certain dance phases generally marked these events (De Martino 1961a). At the outset, the tarantata would lie prostrate on a white sheet stretched out on the ground until a musical note performed by a small orchestra of musicians moved her into action, bringing her desperation to the surface, into her moves, screams, gestures and grimaces. Her head would beat from side to side and her back arch upward. She would roll over and over and eventually jump up to execute elements of the pizzica pizzica in an ever more frantic manner, before spinning on the spot and collapsing to the ground. Just a short break would provide some rest before another dance cycle was resumed with the same dancer.

The crises of the tarantate involved symptoms associated with a range of physiological rhythms, ranging from the lethargic (listlessness, drowsiness, paralysis) to the hyperactive (convulsions, trembling, shaking), all of which may be seen to be out of sync with 'healthy' bodily rhythms of the heart, pulse, metabolism or respiration.[24] In the ritual context, the effects of the tarantula's poison were summoned up through audio, visual, kinaesthetic and olfactory stimuli, such as incessant rhythms, rapid movements, colourful ribbons or wild flowers. The afflicted was stimulated to express and accentuate her crisis, to become and enact all that which the tarantula, as an indigenous element of the Salentine fauna, was seen to embody. Her crisis became an integral part of her cure.[25] It was made tangible, audible, visible and accessible to the senses, providing scope for the transformation of experiences and self-perceptions, in individual, social and political terms. A cure was achieved when the individual treated felt better, when a visceral sense of well-being, of presence or 'kinaesthetic attentiveness' (Desjarlais 1996: 145) manifested itself through vitality, spontaneity and perceptive responsiveness.[26] How this happened and whether it still does were the questions that took me to southern Italy.

Tracking Down the Spider: Research Techniques and Intentions

I first came to the Salento in late August 1996 on a brief holiday. On the highway to Lecce, the Salentine capital, an Apulian friend assured me that we were heading for the most beautiful part of Italy. My unspoken expectations, merging hearsay of tarantism and stereotypes of southern Italy, grew with his enthusiasm for showing us a region of which the defects and hardships were skilfully dispersed into jokes, clearing the windscreen beyond surface appearances to that considered worthy of identification. In the early evening, we walked through the streets of Lecce, with their yellow street lights transforming the baroque frills of white stone buildings and endless churches into stunning shadows. I was struck by the numerous votive corners with religious statues, glowing light bulbs and flowers set into house walls; by crowds promenading the streets in high-street fashions; by designer stores flanking workshops of artisans, cobblers or bicycle menders, tucked away in windowless basements below street level.

We camped for a couple of days near the Baia dei Turchi, the bay of the Turks, just north of the Adriatic port of Otranto: a major source of conflict by 2006, between local environmentalists and entrepreneurs responsible for illegally constructing the foundations of a summertime bar on this spot.[27] The coastline here was a dazzling turquoise, alternating cliffs and sandy patches, scarcely dotted with sunbathers, occasional fishermen and carelessly discarded rubbish. Like many parts of the Salento, Otranto speaks of a history of foreign domination[28]: the fortified city centre, with its castle rendered famous by Horace Walpole's (1764) gothic tale, conserves a cathedral with a millennium-old mosaic floor of intertwined mythical and biblical figures and a chapel of skulls and bones commemorating the martyrs of the fifteenth-century Turkish assault.[29]

One afternoon we drove to Galatina, trade fair town and home to the chapel of St Paul, patron saint of the tarantula's victims.[30] Thanks to the apostle's protection, this municipality has always been ascribed

9

immunity to the spider's bite and no cases of tarantism have, apparently, been registered among its citizens. In August 1996, the town sign was punctured by two holes recalling bullet shots. The fields around were burnt black with ashes. Industrial sites marked the periphery, while the historical town centre appeared abandoned. It was three o'clock in the afternoon and the heat had driven everyone but a few phantom strollers off the streets. To our astonishment the local library was open and the director kindly furnished me with a number of texts on tarantism. Curiosity threw me into anthropological mode: hands and feet complementing poor language skills, antennae stretched to a maximum. We moved to the central piazza stretching out at the feet of the main church's elaborate façade.

In my mind, the pavement stones came alive in black and white moving images: films I had seen of the tarantate, brides of St Paul, dressed in white, running in wild circles on this very square, driven by vehement impulses, screaming in high-pitched voices, terrorizing spectators and attacking those dressed in bright colours [see Fig. 1.2]. A clergyman crossed our tracks and cars circled around us like a traffic island in the square centre, as the priest's tales of horse-drawn carriages bringing desperate men and women to St Paul's shrine, mixed with his greetings to passers-by. The tiny chapel remained closed all year, except for three days at the end of June when the town patrons were celebrated and numerous pilgrims came to its threshold. On rare occasions, the doors were opened out of season to calm those seeking St Paul's blessing. For us, too, the keys were sought out and we were taken into the tiny space long since deconsecrated by the Catholic Church. The air was thick, lacking ventilation, suggestive of emotional outbursts lived and exorcised between these walls. In the years to come, I was to return often, following up old stories, observing new ones.

Yet, beyond the imposing coastline, I failed to see the predicted beauty of this region. What struck me were the pale, sometimes lifeless, colours: yellow grass, grey stone-ridden earth, silver olive groves, a late-summer landscape drained of moisture. No strong distinctions caught the eye beyond cement structures of unfinished buildings or abandoned farmhouses, distorted out of focus by the heat. There was no record of the colourful spectacle springtime blossoms create each year. Nevertheless, something seduced me to undertake fieldwork here, in this part of southern Italy.

My point of departure to look at the tarantula's music and dance was a strong curiosity to find out more about this tradition, exploring the labels of normality and madness cloaked in varying explanations of affliction and cure. The tarantate of southern Italy have variously been branded as mad, hysterical, psychologically unstable, exhibitionistic; the connotations of 'not being credible' associated with these classificatory tags marked the lives of many. These views, however, contradict the respect accorded to them by others, who emphasize their access to unique insights, 'something like white magic', due to their relation to the tarantula.[31]

This range of opinions and the motivations that lay at their foundation intrigued me. Often I was asked: 'Do you believe in the tarantula?' My response was that, in some way and over a considerable time span, tarantism had been seen to work. It would not have lasted for centuries if its effects had not been considered and experienced as beneficial. Inevitably, however, the notion of efficacy depends on the criteria applied. Tarantism has worked both to liberate and to oppress. It has been a channel of release and resolution when there was no other perceived way out. In these terms, it has been safety valve and golden cage all in one. Nevertheless, for the purposes of anthropological research it is valuable to accept the belief system of tarantism as one possible reality, as one possible epistemology of healing. For those afflicted by the tarantula spider, its poison was real in its effects even in the absence of an actual bite. Apparent contradictions in empirical terms dissolved as different notions of reality came into play.

The anthropologist moves between these, not always without risk, open to various ways of reading the world. At the outset of my fieldwork a professor in theatre history at the University of Lecce advised me as follows, touching on the subtle divide between taking part, in order to understand, and keeping apart, so as not to lose touch with the ground under one's feet:

Tarantism is a phenomenon made up of a million folds. If you unfold it, explain it, it won't exist any more. It is not a fixed or bounded system. Instead, it is something dynamic, constantly being translated and transformed. You must focus on the relations between things. In order to relate, you have to open up, break and diffuse your own boundaries. If something does not finish, it can be transformed. You need to consider how things speak to each other, how objects and people play together. And you too have to be prepared to open up, to engage with others, to break your own ways of thinking. Our way of seeing the world appears to be the most efficient for our current lives. But, this does not mean that there are no other ways of seeing the world.[32]

This book does not claim to explain the tarantate's rituals or the contemporary pizzica scene. Instead, it strives to paint an impressionistic picture of the manifold facets of everyday life within which the notes and steps of the tarantula's music and dance came and come alive. With this intention, it portrays both unique lives and dynamic cultural contexts. It can never do justice to the whole – there are many musicians I have never talked to, many dancers I have never met, audio-visual recordings and written documents I have not located – but it can begin to provide a sense of what it meant and means to live in this part of Italy.

It is important to stress, moreover, that this research may be seen to address the lives of only a minority of Salentines[33] today: by 2006, the number of (ex)tarantate was estimated to be no more than five or six, while in 1998 fifteen to twenty were still said to be alive.[34] Widespread opinion completely denies their existence, since none are believed to be practising rituals any longer. What is more, despite the crowds attracted by pizzica concerts, those linking this music and dance (still or again) to a therapeutic potential (variously defined) are limited in number and often contradicted by more popular views, defining this contemporary boom exclusively in terms of entertainment, politics, tourism, commercialization and questions of identity. Finally, there are many who have had enough of all the buzz around the spider and are likely to roll their eyes when yet another pizzica is played.

Initially, when I came to the Salento, I did not know whether it would still be possible to find anyone who had lived through the ordeals attributed to the tarantula. At the same time, I had no idea that the music and dance once associated with this healing tradition were about to boom beyond anyone's expectations. Before I knew it, my footnotes on this aspect turned into entire chapters. My research, in turn, gradually extended over a decade (1996–2008), involving various periods of long-term residence in the Salento. I was always based in Lecce, but travelled throughout the surrounding area pursuing two main tracks of investigation: one focused on researching the historical healing ritual of tarantism and the other following the spotlight on contemporary performances of the tarantula's music and dance.

Tracking down tarantism involved background research on existing publications in academic writing, local media and literature, as well as on audio-visual media, Internet resources, films, photographs and sound recordings. It implied participating at conferences and other encounters (discussions, book presentations, photographic exhibitions) organized on this topic by the University of Lecce and other institutions, as well as cultural associations in the Salento and elsewhere. Most importantly this fieldwork allowed me to hear the stories of those who have lived with the tarantula: in their own lives, families or towns. Almost everybody had an anecdote to tell.

Researching the world of neo-tarantism allowed more scope for direct involvement. Particularly in the summer months, celebrations (religious festivals, fairs and concerts) associated with the pizzica provided the most valuable occasions for gathering insights through impromptu conversations, observing and participating. I learnt to dance the pizzica pizzica, but never quite, despite endless generous demonstrations, caught the hang of the tambourine, virtuoso instrument in today's pizzica world. I attended performances of many of the music groups specializing in the pizzica, followed different courses aimed at transmitting its steps and rhythms, as well as rehearsals and tours of the group Arakne Mediterranea, directed by the late Giorgio Di Lecce, while interviews about the current Salentine music scene provided more focused information.

Dancing the pizzica and actively participating in concert settings brought up key lines of enquiry guiding this research. It also evokes a question ethnomusicologists Gregory Barz and Timothy Cooley (1997) posit as central to a 'new ethnography': 'What do we see when we acknowledge the shadows we cast in the field? What do we hear, smell and taste?' A focus not only on representing but also on 'doing' and 'knowing' in fieldwork aims to convey a sense of what it means 'to be in the world musically' and, I would add, 'to be in the world choreographically'. As Barz and Cooley (1997: 208) point out: 'Ethnography in this sense becomes an integral part of the translation of experience, an extension of the field performance, and ultimately a form of performance writing.' It acknowledges the agency of the ethnographer both in and out of the field as 'chasing whatever is hidden behind the shadows he or she casts in the field' (ibid.: 209).

13

This book too, becomes a dance with shadows, with inevitable limitations coming to the surface.

Five of these limitations stand out. First and foremost, I myself have never seen a ritual of tarantism. Instead, I rely on the memories of others, on what their voices convey, always, inevitably, filtered by time and their, as well as my own, perceptions. At the same time, each story can be played against others and cross-checked against the large quantity of historical documents available, so as to guarantee the maximum possible reliability of the data presented.

Secondly, the approach taken may be seen to achieve no more than documenting the last vestiges of tarantism. Such criticism needs to be taken seriously. The temptation of continuity is highly seductive, as historian Peregrine Horden (2000, 2003) warns, and it would be reductive to consider the small number of remaining tarantate as representative of 'tarantism', seeing that not only its protagonists but also understandings of the term tarantism itself have undergone and continue to undergo incessant changes.

Thirdly, this study compares the tarantula's music and dance in highly different performative contexts, which are difficult to pigeonhole or define in themselves and, according to some, completely incomparable. 'The pizzica today', as many Salentines would insist, 'has nothing to do with tarantism, although a process of bastardization between the two has taken place.'[35] Motivations for performing may be seen as utterly split between the diverging aims of healing (in the past) and hedonism, including tourism (today). Moreover, past and present dances may be differentiated according to the categories of ritual versus theatre or spectacle, bringing into relief the manifold problems associated with the use of these categories.[36] Yet the tarantula's thread weaves through both contexts, revealing how its meanings change not only in time, but also on a case by case basis, without, however, implying proof of common descent.

Fourthly, my data inevitably are conditioned not only by my own view, but also by the people I have come to know. Generally speaking, I have had more contact with groups who led the 1990s revitalization and am less familiar with more recently formed bands.[37]

Finally, ethical issues emerge, since this study addresses sensitive material related to affliction and suffering, which risks becoming sensational and commercial in a context that celebrates the pizzica and has turned research on tarantism into a fashion. This brings to mind a question guiding anthropologist Valentine Daniel's (1996: 3) work on violence: 'How to give an account of ... shocking events, without giving in to the desire to shock?' As a consequence, I have opted to use pseudonyms in a few cases in which I was not given express consent to use real names, and trust that those who would have liked to be mentioned by name will empathize with this decision. It allows this research to be made accessible to those whose cultural identities are addressed, while at the same time respecting the individual identity of those who have entrusted me with their views and experience.[38]

Crisis, Celebrity and Celebration: Contextualizing Salentine Tarantulas

A focus on process and performativity guides this exploration of bygone tarantism rituals and today's pizzica events as cultural forms of expression for articulating the highs and lows of daily life. It suggests that, just as in the days of the tarantate, dynamics of projection and identification continue to mark the worlds of those engaging with the spider's image today: whereas the tarantate had to identify with their afflicting spider in order to evoke its presence and then pacify or expel it, Salentines today use the music and dance that once drove out poison to create an identity distinguishing themselves from others, be these northern Italians, Europeans more generally, tourists, participants in the 'world music' scene or yet others. Some Salentines speak of having the pizzica in their blood, creating a sense of community defined on the basis of musical DNA, seen to render them unique (Gala 2002a, b; Pizza 2002a, b).[39]

Such a 'self' versus 'other' contrast may express more subtle dynamics characterizing contemporary Western society: fears of dissolving boundaries, fleeting points of reference, and a gaping meaninglessness of existence more generally.[40] Although such dissolving boundaries may equally further a sense of community among humanity at large, well-being may be jeopardized by crises expressed under new labels today – stress, depression, nervous breakdown or addictions – or fatalistic and fanatical points of view. In such situations of distress, the tarantula's music and dance can (but not necessarily do) intervene, by transforming perceptions of the self, others and reality at large. Spider dances draw attention, moreover, to motivations for and experiences of performing beyond explicitly choreographic or musicological criteria, bringing into focus ethnomusicological and other literature on the relation between music and identity (Stokes 1994; Feld 2000; Connell and Gibson 2003).

Identity has been widely defined in opposition to alterity, a dichotomy that anthropologists have carefully deconstructed, in an effort to 'discard any essentialited notion of difference, to eschew any over emphasis on identity as sameness and to resist any temptation to moralize about "othering"' (Gingrich 2004: 15).[41] Anthropological studies have highlighted how any group's apparently consolidated identity may involve a cross-boundary struggle for control and contestations from within the group, challenging the absolute character of discourses on identity and the existence of defining boundaries that are not only a matter of degree but also of kind (Cohen 2000: 1–2). 'Wherever we look in the world, people are fighting back in a struggle for identities which they can regard as more sensitive to themselves, rejecting self-denying generalisation and subordination to collective categories' (Cohen 1994: 177). This has led to sensitive and complex debates on rights to identity, and who defines such identities, in the face of imposed matrices of perception.

The French-Lebanese writer Amin Maalouf (2000) stresses how a widespread habit of thought assumes that we have one major affiliation defining our identity. This, he warns, is a simplistic recipe for massacres. He calls for a new concept of identity not based on the denial of the 'self' versus the denial of the 'other', but recognizing instead that each and everyone's identity is complex, unique and irreplaceable – a minority in itself. Current perceptions of phenomena such as 'globalization' inevitably reinforce a need for identity, while at the same time they potentially hold the key to a new perspective emphasizing the common identity of humankind.[42] Global media play a key role in this context.

Morley and Robins (1995) have considered the media's implications in reimagining a contemporary Europe 'without frontiers'. Anxieties provoked by shifting and dissolving boundaries and points of reference, leading to a sense of disorientation and loss of control, are soothed by 'calls for the pure (if mythic) certainties of the "old traditions"' (ibid.: 8).

Without discrediting mass migrations in the past, being European (as well as global citizenship more generally) increasingly demands juggling continental, national and regional identities in one. It implies negotiating with and commitment to that which is considered to be different. It implies a world with increasingly porous boundaries, 'an intensification of global interconnectedness' (Inda and Rosaldo 2002: 2), characterized by multiple understandings and realities of 'globalization' with its 'crisscrossing flows and intersecting systems of meanings' (ibid.: 26).

Music, as one of many performance genres, is a further key player in this context. 'World music' – a prime label for the tarantula's music and dance – may be seen as 'today's dominant signifier of a triumphant industrialization of global sonic representation' (Feld 2000: 146).[43] Music is more often than not seen to epitomize places, fostering not only marketing strategies, relying on claims to the 'traditional', 'authentic' and 'original', but also music tourism (Connell and Gibson 2003). Meanwhile, spatial coordinates assign credibility and money value to music. Music and place reciprocally define each other (Stokes 1994). The pizzica, for example, draws its contemporary power from associations with historical tarantism, frequently seen to be rooted in Salentine territory. Attempts at deconstructing such links challenge music's selling power, its mystic appeal and spiritual magnetism. Steven Feld (2000: 154) points to 'world music', moreover, not only as a discourse, but also as a fundamental zone of activities and representation involving 'intersubjective clashes for musicians, recordists, industry players, journalists and academics'.

The varying intentions of these diverse actors come into play and conflict, raising accusations of cultural commoditization and theft reminiscent of those expressed in the face of tourism (Kirtsoglou and Theodossopoulos 2004), echoed in much of the literature on this topic. Some stress that 'the tourist is a kind of contemporary pilgrim, seeking authenticity in other "times" and other "places" away from that person's everyday life' (Urry 2000: 9). Such views are reinforced by recent studies on pilgrimage and healing showing how typical motivations of curing afflictions, whether of a physical or spiritual nature, are complemented in the animated field of modern-day pilgrimages with those of quests for identity, for 'reassembling the self', and interpersonal connection (Badone and Roseman 2004;

17

Basu 2004; Coleman and Eade 2004; Dubisch and Winkelman 2005). Others see tourist aspirations as less enchanted, as thriving on 'pseudo-events' (Boorstin 1961) and, more significantly, have problematized the notion of authenticity as existing not only in various stages (MacCannell 1999) but also as a negotiable and constantly changing point of reference (Chambers 1999). This multifaceted picture provides a backdrop for a look at the contemporary music and dance scene in the Salento.

Mutations in the tarantula's music and dance show how experiences of the self both mould and are moulded by the props, actions and choices of protagonists. Definitions and diagnoses of performers reveal culturally specific self-perceptions, including views of affliction and well-being. Research in medical anthropology and performance studies (including anthropological approaches) provides useful guidelines in this respect. Medical anthropologists have emphasized the cultural specificity of health or illness (Kleinman 1980; Young 1982; Helman 1984) and the socially constructed nature of the human body (Blacking 1977; Turner 1992; Lock 1993; Csordas 2002). Work on theatre and performance studies, meanwhile, has problematized Western notions of 'theatre', 'dance' and 'performance', searching for cross-culturally applicable categories in order to discover what performance can reveal about society (Turner 1982; Schechner 1985; Barba and Savarese 1991; Beeman 1993; Thomas 2003). Studies on dance have turned attention to embodied cultural practices and individual experience in performance (Peterson Royce 1977, 2004; Hanna 1979; Spencer 1985; Ness 1992; Reed 1998; Farnell 1999; Buckland 1999, 2006; Kaeppler 2000; Dils and Cooper Albright 2001), while ethnomusicologists have fine-tuned our awareness to the importance of music and soundscapes in diverse cultural settings (Merriam 1964; Blacking 1976; Nettl 1983; Myers 1984; Seeger 1987; Feld 1990; Barz and Cooley 1997; Mackinlay et al. 2005).

These studies, together with research in the 'anthropology of the senses' (Stoller 1989; Howes 1992, 2004; Geurtz 2002; Desjarlais 2003; Classen 2005) have prompted medical anthropologists to explore the therapeutic impact of dramatic media in performative contexts (Laderman 1991; Devish 1993; Roseman 1993; Jennings 1995; Laderman and Roseman 1996; Sklar 2001; Sax 2004), as well as notions of embodiment and experience with respect to the curative process (Desjarlais 1992; Csordas 1994, 2002). Recent publications addressing the relation between healing, dance and music have made reference to tarantism, but almost exclusively with regard to its historical forms (Tomlinson 1994; Gouk 2000; Horden 2000, 2003; Del Giudice 2003).

In this context, I regard the tarantula's dance in terms of performance, on the basis of the premise that 'performance enters all domains of human existence in both secular and religious fields; the "dramas of everyday life", as well as the "dramas set apart", i.e., theatre and ritual' (Jennings 1995: 9).[44] Performance practices such as music making and dance viewed in terms of actor training, as a process rather than an end product, imply that ways of using the human organism alternative or complementary to those of daily life are acquired. If the recovery of well-being, meanwhile, is seen in terms of a negotiative process transforming culturally specific notions of affliction into those of well-being and vitality, this means that alternative or complementary ways of perceiving and experiencing the human organism are learned. Acting theories (Artaud 1958; Grotowski 1976; Stanislavski 1980a, b, 1981; Brook 1993, 1998; Schechner 2002) may be drawn upon to show how performance may be used to express the inner experience of a specific character, including that of affliction, in socially accepted terms. In this sense, the actor's experience of theatrical malleability, the potential of moving among many different roles, may both reflect and shape sociocultural upbringing. This correlation may underlie the direct and potentially therapeutic impact of performance practices on the experience of everyday life, taking into account that well-being relates both to the microscopic level of individual health and illness and to the macroscopic level of collective life and social policy (Jennings 1994; Laderman and Roseman 1996; Lock and Scheper-Hughes 1996).

Preview: Summarizing this Book

Part I, Past and Present Spider Webs, sets the scene, showing how the tarantula's cult continues, as it has for centuries, to intrigue Salentines and others alike. On 29 June, St Paul, patron saint of the tarantate, is revered and celebrated. Chapter 1, 'Seeking St Paul', takes a look at festivities in the town of Galatina, pilgrimage site of his devotees, displaying the contradictory and complex ways in which the tarantula's myth and music have been both preserved and reinvented. Chapter 2, 'Webs through Time', places this first-hand scenario in historical perspective. A review of the rich and varied literature on tarantism and its origins shows how this ritual tradition not only represents but also disputes specific conceptions of human nature, society and reality dominating various stages of European history.

Part II, The Spider's Cult Today, provides ethnographic detail, revealing how the spider remains a common denominator while its meanings vary greatly. In the contemporary Salento, tarantism and neo-tarantism exist side by side. Chapter 3, 'Curing Myths and Fictive Cures', reveals how in its traditional, curative form, the tarantula's dance has died out with rare exceptions carefully concealed from the public eye. For a very few elderly Salentines devotion to the tarantula and St Paul continues to be the only way out of their misery. However, according to the majority of the Salento's inhabitants, tarantism has, thankfully, been eradicated and remains nothing but a myth of the past, of which only the music and dance are worth preserving. In its novel, reformulated sense, the spider's cult is gaining new fans daily, while its concerts are attracting crowds in the thousands, as Chapter 4, 'Ads and Antidotes', confirms. The myth, music and dance of tarantism inevitably serve contemporary purposes: some seek experiences of 'magic' (variously described), or expressive forms accentuating personal virtuosity. Yet others desire a cultural source of identity and orientation, often reflected in tourist ads and media hype. At the same time, spider dances have become a means through which to take a position and demand change, be it political, ecological or other. Varying degrees of conflict emerge from looking at the motives that drive participants to perform and applaud the pizzica today. Chapter 5, 'Sensing Identities and Well-being', moves on to look at personal stories behind the buzz continuing to bring alive discourses of recovering well-being.

Part III, From Ritual to Limelight, involves an analysis of ambiguities and contradictions that bring to the fore subtle social dynamics and power structures impeding or fostering well-being. 'Dances with spiders' in the Salento implies both performances addressing life crises and festive entertainments shimmering in the limelight. Chapter 6, 'SpiderWoMen Transfixed', explores what criteria characterize the perceptions and afflictions of old and new tarantati, and questions how these relate to views of human nature and reality, as well as treatment choices more generally. Chapter 7, 'Tarantula Threads and Showbiz Airs', takes a look at places, times, props and techniques making up the complex choreographies of past and present spider dances. In the past, no cure was possible unless the tarantula's thread, that stimulus which persuaded the tarantate to dance, was found. Today, a concert's success depends on detecting the appropriate air or music compelling bystanders to take part and applaud. Beyond financial backing, networking and good technological resources, this requires not merely technical virtuosity, but above all the mutual interaction of performers and their willingness to surrender to the music. Chapter 8, 'SpiderWoMen Transformed', focuses on personal experiences of the tarantula's music and dance in the context of performance circles ascribed 'magic' qualities. It considers how rhythmic interaction can sensitize performers' abilities to access vitality and choices promoting well-being, thereby providing a playground to move beyond the afflicted victim role to that of a creative 'choreographer'.

The Conclusion, Chapter 9, 'Dancing Beyond Spiders', draws together the key threads of this study. Considerations of tarantism and its modern developments suggest that afflictions associated with the tarantula's cult in the past persist under new labels today. It emphasizes the need for a greater sensitivity towards the potential value of certain human conditions, which may be pathologized according to Western psychiatric categories, while being inherently transformative and therapeutic if safeguarded by a network of social support and meaning. What is more, the Salento today reveals how performance arts, such as the pizzica, can effect changes in the perception of ourselves, others and reality at large. This transformative capacity has the potential not only to distress and divide but also to heal and unite.

Notes

1. Hundertwasser Haus, Vienna.

2. The two terms 'tarantism' and 'tarantolism' may be used interchangeably, although the former is more frequently heard in the Salento and hence also adopted in this study. The notion of cult is used here in a broad sense to indicate both a body of organized cultural practices and beliefs shared by a group of people (tarantism in its traditional forms), and a phenomenon that is popular or fashionable among a devoted group of enthusiasts (the contemporary revitalization of the tarantula's music and dance).

3. The tarantella dance characteristic of southern Italy is known for its skipping steps and lively 3/8 or 6/8 rhythms, often in accelerating tempo. There are many regional variations, including the Apulian *pizzica* or *pizzica pizzica*, which is today largely associated with the Salento. Interestingly, the term tarantella is rarely used by Salentines to refer to the pizzica, but features in other well-known contexts: as concert pieces, such as Chopin's opus 43; as a theatrical prop in Henrik Ibsen's *A Doll's House*; and, more recently, as a *tarantallegra* jinx in J.K. Rowling's *Harry Potter and the Chamber of Secrets* (1998).

4. I use the feminine singular and plural forms of these two synonyms to talk about the victims of the tarantula in the past. Although this goes against the conventions of Italian grammar, particularly when speaking about plural forms which also include men, this choice is motivated by the fact that most of those afflicted were women. Generally speaking, both terms (*tarantata/tarantato* or *tarantolata/tarantolato*) and both feminine and masculine plural forms (*tarantate* or *tarantati*) are used interchangeably, depending on the sex of the victim referred to or the preferences of the speaker. When talking about the contemporary context, I choose the term modern or new (*nuovi*) tarantati, to refer to those engaging with the symbol of the tarantula today, as both men and women are involved.

5. I use the terms 'revitalized' or 'revitalization' in this study, following Tak (2000: 209), to avoid the term 'revival', which may be misread as a return to a previously existing situation, discounting the impact of changes in the political economy.

6. I use the expression 'tarantula's music and dance' to refer to Salentine music, including especially but not exclusively the pizzica, associated both with past rituals of tarantism and the contemporary revitalization movement. Although this expression risks conflating past and present performances, furthering assumptions of continuity, the notion of 'tarantula' is taken here as a multi-purpose denominator shaped by and shaping diverse, eclectic and potentially contradictory choices, intentions and performances. The pizzica is commonly described as *musica popolare* in the

22

Salento, a term indicating traditional musical genres that are orally transmitted within a specific ethnic region or group, not to be confused with 'pop music' or commercial genres of music with a widespread and often short-term appeal characterizing Westernized and modernized societies. The term 'folk music' is avoided so as to focus on the specificity of Salentine music, while at the same time acknowledging the vast and varied repertoires characterizing the music and dance scene of the Salento.

7. In this study, the geographical range of the Salento is largely taken to be the Provincia di Lecce – reaching from a few towns just north of the capital to the very southern tip of the peninsula – although the Salento is generally seen to comprise the three provinces of Lecce, Brindisi and Taranto. This choice is based on the fact that the area around Lecce has been most strongly (but not exclusively) exposed to the revitalization of the pizzica and thus is also largely where I undertook my research.

8. The *Latrodectus tredecim guttatus*, also known as Mediterranean black widow, malmignatte or karakurt spider, is found throughout the Mediterranean region. It is characterized by thirteen red spots on its otherwise black dorsal abdomen (hence its Latin name for 'thirteen spots'). Its bite is venomous to humans unlike that of the *Lycosa tarantula*, or wolf spider, which is essentially harmless. See also, Chapter 6, 'Diagnosing Spiders: Identifying Tarantula Cases'.

9. 'Bites by widow spiders often are initially painful, but sometimes are not felt. The local dermal reaction is minimal, usually consisting of little more than an area of erythema (redness) around the bite site, which disappears within several hours; no tissue necrosis occurs following bites by widow spiders. A potent neurotoxin in the venom induces the disease state latrodectism, which manifests itself with severe muscle cramping and spasms; the cramping usually begins in the large muscle masses of the legs, or the abdomen. The abdomen can exhibit a board-like rigidity, and the pain has been compared to that of acute appendicitis, and to childbirth. Some widow bite victims experience anxiety, profuse sweating, nausea, piloerection (hair standing on end), increased blood pressure, and other unpleasant manifestations. Paralysis, stupor and convulsions, as well as psychological abnormalities may occur in severe cases. Death can occur in a small percentage of cases, particularly when the victim is a small child or elderly person.' Retrieved on 30 September 2007 from http://www.srv.net/~dkv/ hobospider/widows.html.

10. The origin of this term remains, to my knowledge, unclear. I first came across it in conversations with informants on my arrival in the Salento in April 1997. US scholar Luisa Del Giudice writes: 'I believe I coined this term in 1996 to refer, in conversation and in interviews, to the folk revival movement which had as its point of reference historic *tarantismo*. I note

with the passing of the years that it has become a term with a certain currency' (Del Giudice 2005: 219). Others attribute this notion to the French academic George Lapassade, who undertook research in the Salento during the 1980s, or associate it with the sociologist Anna Nacci, author of the books *Tarantismo e neotarantismo* (2001) and *Neotarantismo* (2004).

11. For translations, see De Martino (1966, 1999, 2005). For reviews in English, French and German, see Anon. (1967); Cassin (1962); De Martino (1961b). In this book, general considerations regarding De Martino's work on tarantism refer to his original 1961 study in Italian (1961a). Specific references to and quotations from this work refer to Dorothy Zinn's 2005 translation.

12. Economic underdevelopment and unemployment are widespread in the Salento, as in much of southern Italy. In the 1960s and 1970s, severe poverty led a large proportion of the working population to emigrate to northern Italy or northern Europe. Many jobs continue to be characterized by unreliable incomes and little, if any, social security, despite modernization in terms of technology, communication, transport and, especially, tourism.

13. This fact is reminiscent of ethnomusicologist Anthony Seeger's (1987: 25–51) admonition regarding 'categories of orality', including both song and speech forms, highlighting the importance of looking at both music and dance in relation to other art forms, as 'everything is always partly defined by what it is not' (ibid.: 25). Various types of pizzica songs exist in parallel to religious songs (funeral laments, hymns, Christmas and Lent songs), songs of work and protest, lullabies and rhymes, as well as narrative songs. Dances of the pizzica, moreover, exist today in a context in which village squares host events with musicians and dancers singing and stepping to all kinds of rhythms, particularly during summer nights: from mazurka, polka or waltz, to synchronized group dances and Latin American styles or the less prescribed motions and words of rap and rave fans, not to mention the overflowing open-air discos with their multiple and varied dance floors, dominated by techno and house beats.

14. Dance ethnologist Giuseppe Gala has also coined new labels to speak about the contemporary *neopizzica* or *emopizzica* as he calls it: *slow-pizzica, trance-pizzica, energico-pizzica, techno-pizzica* (Gala 2002a: 109–53). Maurizio Nocera, meanwhile, speaks of the *pizzica di sofferenza*, the pizzica of suffering, a term he heard various tarantate use to describe their healing dances (Lecce, 1 April 2006).

15. Daniele Vigna explains, for example, that while in the pizzica pizzica the 'triplet is characteristic, in the scherma circle it is the strong beat which provides the base' (Monaco 2006: 89).

16. See Gala's website: www.taranta.it/pizzica.html. Gala also emphasizes that other dances need to be kept in mind, such as the *scotis* or *quadriglia* (Galatina, Estadanza, July 2002).

17. The north Italian region of Piedmont, for example, is known for its sword dances in San Giorio, Limone, Giaglione and Venaus (Val di Susa). See Galanti (1950: 7).

18. This confusion in terminology has raised criticism among those who view it as a misrepresentation of historical facts and a repercussion of the widespread popularity of large-scale media events such as the annual Night of the Tarantula concert.

19. Archivio della Curia Arcivescovile, Lecce, *Giudicati matrimoniali,* 'Tra Francesco Ardito e Catarina Russo', no. 891.

20. Interestingly, to this day, someone who cannot stay still may be described in Italian as a person who has the tarantula (*ha la tarantola*) (Naselli 1951: 222).

21. In his *Lettere dal carcere,* Letters from Prison, dated 11 April 1927, Gramsci (1965) describes the scherma in the barracks of Castellammare.

22. For television and cinematographic features (both documentary and fiction) on the pizzica pizzica, see Stegmueller and Koeplin (1992); Bevilacqua (1995); Canizzaro (2001, 2003) Daudy (2001); Marengo (2005); Pisanelli (2005); Colopi and Giagnotti (2008). For a feature on the scherma, see Fersini (2005). For features on the pizzica tarantata, see Carpitella (1960); Miscuglio et al. (1981); Mingozzi (1982); Durante (1989); Winspeare (1989, 1994, 2000); Santoro and Durante (1993); Gallone (2006). This list cannot claim to be complete, nor does it account for numerous videos and DVDs produced on this topic.

23. Links emerge between the pizzica di cuore and other dances of lure, coax and escape, such as the Cuban and Puerto Rican guagnanco, an Afro-Cuban form of rumba (Friedman 1978). Inevitable connections to the flamenco come to mind: another seductive dance in the Mediterranean context on the cusp of Europe, on the silk trade route, connected with North and West Africa through trade and conquest and with Gypsies on the move between Eastern and Western Europe, thereby combining Muslim, Gypsy, Indian and African influences (Comerford Peters and Schreiner 1990; Washabaugh 1996). Likewise, the tango with its embodiment of sensuality, eroticism and competition provides further parallels (Savigliano 1995; Taylor 1998; Archetti 1999). Meanwhile, the scherma brings to mind associations with various martial arts (Zarrilli 2000; Jones 2002), as well as the Brazilian capoeira (Lowell Lewis 1992; Downey 2005), which presents another combat dance and channel of expression for grievances that could not be expressed otherwise. Although essentially unarmed, dancers to this day use knives and machetes (as well as the more recent urban addition of razors) in their exhibitions (Lowell Lewis 1992: 41).

24. Beyond the possible (but atypical) local effects of actual bites, visible as red and swollen punctures on the skin, the tarantate revealed a series of general reactions: vomiting, sweating, stomach, muscular and heart pains, nausea,

vertigo, fainting, headaches, hyperventilation, cyanosis, dyspnoea, weak pulse, fever, extreme cold, numbness, delirium, loss of appetite, sleepiness, insomnia, fatigue, paralysis, convulsions and trembling (Russell 1979: 410–11). Extremes of bodily and rhythmic mobility or immobility stood out. Behavioural symptoms were equally varied, including depression, a strong sense of fear and anguish, weeping, laughing, permissive sexual conduct, as well as jumping, dancing and singing as symptoms overlapped with treatment techniques.

25. See Kleinman (1980), Helman (1984), Sargent and Johnson (1996), Nichter and Lock (2002) for debates in medical anthropology on the use of terminology associated with affliction and cure. See Mathews and Izquierdo (2008) for anthropological perspectives on well-being.

26. Elements of the tarantate's rituals may be reminiscent of Robert Desjarlais's (1996: 160) description of the healing performances of Yolmo shamans in Nepal as rejuvenating a spiritless body: 'By adding to what a person tastes, sees, touches, hears and imagines, a Yolmo healer jump-starts a physiology.'

27. See www.baiadeiturchi.ilcannochiale.it.

28. If we may reduce 2500 years of local history to a snapshot, the region known as the Salento was inhabited in Antiquity by a variety of peoples: the Messapians, Iapygians, Bruttii and Sallentini. These people remained partly independent of the strong Greek colonies of Magna Graecia, but both the Greeks and the earlier inhabitants fell to the Romans during their expansion in the third century BC. Parts of this Roman-held territory were held by the late Roman and Byzantine rulers while the rest was taken by the Longobards from the north. Brief periods of Arab rule in some sites were followed by Byzantine rule in the ninth century, succeeded by a Norman conquest in the late eleventh century. These were followed by Swabian, Angevin, Aragonese, Spanish, Austrian Hapsburg and Bourbon rulers, with a brief Ottoman Turkish presence in the fifteenth century. The overlapping conquests, with their attendant changes of language, faith, costume and music, helped define the Salento prior to the Unification of Italy in 1861 (see Carducci 1993).

29. In 1480, an Ottoman fleet commanded by general Gedik Ahmed Pasha captured the port city of Otranto. Eight hundred citizens refusing to give up their Christian faith were ruthlessly decapitated. Officially recognized as martyrs by the Church, their remains are exhibited to this day in seven large built-in display cabinets in the city's cathedral.

30. See Rouget (1986), Lapassade (1994, 2001) and De Martino (2005) for a contextualization of tarantism in relation to other cults that have become syncretized with Catholicism, such as the Cuban *santéria*, Brazilian *candomblé* and *umbanda* or Haitian *vodou*.

31. Parabita, 6 August 2001.

32. Melendugno, 25 October 1997.

33. I use the notion 'Salentines' here to refer to the inhabitants of the Salento. However, it is vital to note that this geographically defined group includes highly diverse members in historical, cultural and ethnic terms.

34. Maurizio Nocera, Lecce, 1 April 2006, and Luigi Chiriatti, Lecce, 2 February 1998.

35. Vittorio Marras, Nardò, 9 May 2006.

36. See Beattie (1977), Turner (1982, 1989), Schechner (1985) and Beeman (1993) for discussions on the notions of ritual and theatre.

37. In his book *Opillopillopìopillopillopà: viaggio nella musica popolare salentina 1970–1998*, Luigi Chiriatti (1998) lists the following groups: Aia Noa, Alla Bua, Arakne Mediterranea, Aramirè, Argalìo, Astèria, Avleddha, Canzoniere Grecanico Salentino, Compagnia delle Arti Xanti Jaca, Ghetonìa, I Coreuti, Le Striare, Mascarimirì, Menamenamò, Officina Zoë, Pierpaolo de Giorgi e I Tamburellisti di Torrepaduli, Terra de Menzu, Traudia. By 2007, a number of these groups no longer existed. For most there has been a turnover of group members. Others, such as Gli Ucci, are not mentioned. Meanwhile, other groups have emerged. These include: Acchiatùra, Aioresis, Ajara, Antonio Amato Ensemble, Aria Antica, Aria Corte, Aria Frisca, Arsura, Artenoscia, Athanaton, Briganti di Terra d'Otranto, Conserva Mara, Cotulapete, Criamu, Erva, Gli amici della Taranta, I Calanti, I Figli di Rocco/Manekà, (ex Figli di Rocco), I Scianari, Kalime te Scirocco, Kamafei (ex Kumenei), Kumenei, L'Ardiche, La Taricata, La 'zzamara, Lu Rusciu Nosciu, Macaria, Mays, Nidi d'Arak, Niuri te Sule, Oce te jentu, Original Salento Tarantae, Quista è la strada delle donne belle, Salentorkestra, Salentotò, Santu Pietru cu tutte le chiai, Scazzaca Tarante, Tammurria, Terreneure, Zimbaria. This list does not claim to be comprehensive, as groups may form and break up, nor does it give a sense of respective media coverage and popularity. See also http://www.dmoz.org/World/Italiano/Arte/Musica/ Generi/Etnica_e_Popolare/ Salentina/Artisti/ for a list of group websites.

38. All translations, unless otherwise stated, are my own and I take full responsibility for any misunderstandings. The quotations cited draw from my field notes, transcribed tape recordings and conversations retrieved from memory or elaborated from memos taken during interviews. Where longer interviews are cited, I have at times eliminated the question-answer format and edited the conversation, while aiming to convey the speaker's account with as much immediacy as possible, despite the inevitable limitations of translating from Italian or the Salentine dialect.

39. For anthropological considerations of 'community' in the context of contemporary experiences of social affiliation and solidarity, see Amit (2002); Rapport and Amit (2002).

40. See Cohen (1994); Morris (1994) and Gingrich (2004) for discussions on the notions of 'self' and 'other' on anthropology. See Gupta and Ferguson

(1997) and Rapport (2003) for discussions on the power to define and transform the 'self' in social and cultural contexts that cannot be spatially localized.

41. Gingrich (2004: 14) outlines successive stages in anthropological debates on identity beginning with the 1940s studies on culture and personality, 1960s neo-Marxist approaches, the turn towards self-reflexivity characterizing research in the 1980s, and the 1990s criticism of identity as a notion conceptualized on the basis of static or fixed notions.

42. For a problematization of the notion of globalization, see Inda and Rosaldo (2002).

43. Steven Feld (2000: 146–51) traces the emergence of world music within the global music industry in relation to broader processes of globalization.

44. For a discussion of key problems entailed in the notion of performance, see Schieffelin (1996: 59–84).

Part I
Past and Present
Spider Webs

For centuries, the tarantula ruled the lives and thoughts of many inhabitants of the Salentine peninsula. In present-day Salento, it has woven its way onto the stage. The initial chapter, 'Seeking St Paul', sets the scene, throwing the spotlight on Galatina, trophy town of the spider cult, ever since the interception of the Catholic Church brought the wild dances of the tarantate under the rule of their patron saint St Paul. On 29 June his feast day is celebrated and in 2001 the pilgrimages of old and new tarantati converged here, bringing to the fore contradictions and complexities that have puzzled thinkers for at least seven centuries. Chapter 2, 'Webs through Time', spins this first-hand account into the vicissitudes of European history, unravelling the dynamic links between views of human nature, society and reality at large.

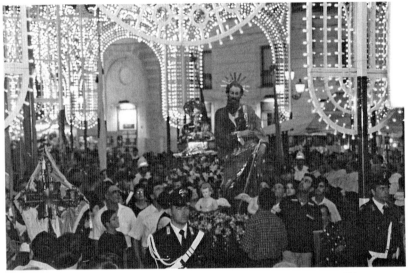

Fig. 1.1 The Festival of St Peter and Paul, Galatina, 28 June 1999. The religious procession with the statue of St Paul and golden bust of St Peter (photo: Karen Lüdtke).

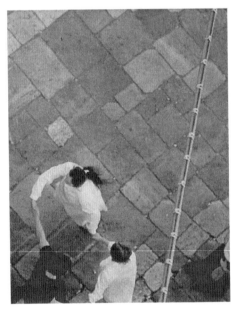 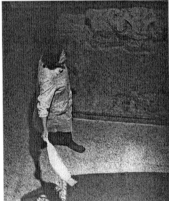

Figs 1.2 and 1.3 The tarantate in Galatina in the early 1970s, dancing on the San Pietro piazza and before the altar inside St Paul's chapel (photos: Paolo Longo).

Chapter 1
Seeking St Paul:
Historical and Contemporary
Enactments

My Saint Paul of the tarantulas,
you who have stung all the girls.
My Saint Paul of Galatina,
give me, and all the others, grace.[1]

I follow Evelina and her family into the main church on the city's
central square, San Pietro piazza, to attend the first mass of this
festival day, as I have ever since we first met in 1998, on the eve of
St Paul's feast day. It takes a little while to get there: on the square,
Evelina's son and his wife explain that Evelina had been fine this
morning, but had gone through her 'troubles' earlier in the year.[2] As
we stand and listen, others gather around to ask a question or two.
Evelina's family speaks openly about this without much ado. In April
and especially in May, they had come to Galatina, to St Paul's chapel,
on several occasions, sometimes even at night. They had been
extremely concerned, fearing Evelina might die, as she would faint
for up to two hours. This was at a time when her grandson was due
to leave to work in the north of Italy and they wondered if her
condition was linked to his coming departure. They had consulted
the family doctor and village priest, but both had advised them to
simply wait, knowing that her pilgrimage to St Paul's chapel in
Galatina would bring relief. It appeared to offer the only source of
alleviation.

It was only 4.30 a.m. when I arrived in Galatina, city of St Peter
and Paul, on 29 June 2001. Festivities mark this feast day and the
cult of St Paul, offshoot of the tarantula's cult, is taking its modern

course, both unique in this cultural context and yet similar to pilgrimages elsewhere (Dubisch and Winkelman 2005). I begin here with an account of what happened in Galatina in the early hours of St Peter and Paul's feast day in 2001. It was the fifth time I had witnessed this event. Never before, however, had I felt so many diverse strands of the tarantula's world come together on one occasion. As old and new tarantati mingled with onlookers and devotees, tensions between what was seen as real or fake emerged, as did the defensiveness and desperation of some appropriating this site for the expression of their personal crises. This occasion brought to the fore key actors and key dynamics composing the worlds of tarantism and neo-tarantism today. The following description of what happened on Galatina's main square on 29 June 2001 makes reference to film footage shot on this very town square in preceding decades, aiming to paint a picture of what has been and is a central stage of the tarantula's cult [see Fig 1.2].

Dances at Galatina: a Crossroads of Old and New Tarantati

Ever since the Catholic Church began to clamp down on dance rituals in the eighteenth century, Paul, protector against poisonous animals, spouse and saviour of the tarantate, has attracted the tarantula's victims to Galatina in their attempts to gain relief. The chapel of St Paul at Galatina has proven to be their most resilient public performance platform. Paul's followers draw their faith from the Bible's account in the New Testament (Acts 28: 3–5), which documents his immunity to a snakebite following a shipwreck on Malta (Montinaro 1996; Ligori et al. 2001). In his travels Paul is said to have passed through Galatina. Nicola Caputo (1741) describes:

> the local belief according to which St Paul landed on the Otranto peninsula and went to the town of Galatina to visit some of its Christians. While there, he bestowed upon a local Christian and his descendants the power to heal those bitten by poisonous animals, by making the sign of the cross over the wound and having the victim drink water from ... the well attached to the house known as *casa di San Paolo*. (Gentilcore 2000: 267)

Only in the eighteenth century was a chapel built inside this house on Via Garibaldi and dedicated to the apostle. Its well was believed to hold healing water, making it a gathering point for the tarantate.[3] By 1959, the well was closed for hygienic reasons and the chapel itself was deconsecrated a few years later. Nevertheless, Paul is the reason behind the small crowd scattered in front of the chapel entrance. Architecturally, little hints at the significance of this doorway. It is identical to the other front portal of the building in which the chapel is set.[4] And yet this inconspicuous site has attracted innumerable pilgrims since its consecration and, what is more, continues to do so.

As I walk into the chapel, I see a starved, strained body crouched on the altar steps below the tapestry of St Paul. It is impossible to identify who this is, but the tense muscles and cramped posture speak for themselves. A man enters the chapel with a guitar, kneels by the shrine and begins to play softly. The sounds are directed towards the distraught body, which collapses onto its left side, moving away from the guitar and indicating for the music to stop. The musician rises and exits, leaving the inert devotee stretched out in front of the altar. Only after some twenty minutes does this young man come to his feet, against what appears to be an enormous weight pulling him down. It is Matteo. I had never seen him before. He leaves the chapel with heavy, tormented strides, as if immune to those around and seemingly not quite present.

Now there is a small group with tambourines and other instruments just outside the chapel restlessly playing pieces of Salentine music. Voices ring out, repeating one of the well-known hymns of the tarantate: 'Santu Paulu meu de le tarante'. Their songs evoke the tarantula, St Paul and Galatina, but are mostly cut short, as if in nervous anticipation of an interruption they would rather pre-empt. There is Annalù Sabetta, known by some as *la striara*, the witch. In her role as 'astrologist, singer, guitar and accordion player, assistant to the tarantate' (Collu 2005: 123), she is – almost imperceptibly – directing the goings-on at the chapel. She calls out to the musicians: 'I'll grant you three, four more minutes.' It is she who has left a bouquet of dried flowers and peacock feathers wrapped in red crêpe paper on the altar. With it, on a white note, there is a dedication: 'For Luigi Stifani'. Annalù explains that she had been in Galatina on this precise day last year, the day that Stifani, famous musician of the tarantate, had died (Stifani 2000; Inchingolo 2003). 'It is significant', she adds, 'that he died on this very day!' This final passage of his life, too, is seen as marked by a link to the tarantula. Annalù is not the only

33

one to identify omens in significant coincidences: in the past, the diagnoses of the tarantate, too, were often based on haphazard encounters with poisonous animals or St Paul, seen to be causative incidents for their afflictions.

A young man approaches Annalù: 'You're a witch, aren't you?' She responds with a laugh, theatrically mocking herself without giving a clear reply: 'Ooooh, yes, I fly!' and her arms swoop up and down in winged motions. Then, she steps out of the chapel and from its threshold, stretches up both arms, directing her attention to the group of young musicians and repeatedly closing her hands into fists. They oblige her gesture and, reluctantly, stop playing.

It begins to rain. Not so distant lightning and thunder set the scene. I stand sheltered under the eaves talking to photographer Fernando Bevilacqua, in his fifties and fervent supporter of local musicians and artists. I'm not surprised to see him here. As we talk, Matteo, moving uneasily around the square, approaches Fernando, interrupting our conversation: 'Even the skies have heard my plea!' Fernando seconds his interpretation: 'If somebody wants something strongly enough, things happen.' Matteo welcomes the rain, the water, while Fernando draws a connection beyond coincidence, perhaps evoking the purifying and cooling qualities of these drops.

Apart from the hum of some thirty people and various video cameras hovering around the chapel entrance, the streets of Galatina are only just beginning to wake up. A rubbish van or two empty dustbins. Cleaners sweep around market stalls, scooping up the dirty traces of the previous night's celebrations. The first vendors, having spent the night behind their stands closed in by canvas blinds, begin to stretch and surface for a coffee in a nearby bar, open early for festive profits. The street lights still throw shadows onto the piazza and the zone carved out by those who have come for St Paul's sake is randomly criss-crossed by others who are oblivious to this space or simply tolerant of it. Cars pass by the chapel, some with partygoers returning home from the previous night's disco, unaware of the hush their passing sends through the small crowd. Will their car stop in front of the chapel doorway? Someone is clearly being expected.

To the citizens of Galatina, this occasion must appear mild and harmless in comparison to not so long ago. Many tell vivid accounts of what happened here in their lifetimes, in the twentieth century. Some tarantate, I was told, came to Galatina on foot, many by carriage and, in later years, by bus or car. Their symptoms often worsened in anticipation of this journey. Some fell into a crisis on departure from their homes. Others saw their crises reappear as they crossed the gates of Galatina. Some stopped here to urinate, expelling bodily fluids as they drew closer to the abode of their celestial husband, St Paul: perhaps a way of providing release from the agitation of coming once again face to face with their fate?

Other tarantate collapsed as they arrived at the chapel of St Paul. Some eyewitnesses report that it was as if the venue itself and the presence of other tarantate created a contagious reaction, which caused the crises of the newly arrived to re-emerge. 'I've been terrified at times to come here,' says Evelina's daughter-in-law. 'Other tarantate seemed to go crazy, shrieking about and jumping around on the altar.'[5] Many performed frantic rounds on San Pietro piazza in front of the small chapel, at times attacking the crowds, infuriated by photographers and cameramen, many of whom took refuge on strategic rooftops and balconies. Everyone who grew up in Galatina knew better than to wear bright clothes or shiny objects on the days the tarantate came to town. Too many had fallen victim to their assaults. Today, these are stories people love to tell. Often it was a bright shirt or dress, red or yellow in particular, or a watch catching the sunlight, which attracted the tarantate's vexed attention and left the terrified owners escaping for their lives, so as not to be left standing on the square, as had happened to others, watchless or, worse still, stripped naked.[6] Intriguingly enough, red is also the colour marking the dorsal abdomen of the European black widow, one of the spider types held responsible for the tarantate's plight.

Verbal assaults still mark the morning of 29 June 2001. 'Andate via! Andate via borghesi!' (Go away! Go away, bourgeois!) The angry shouts of Matteo ring out from where he is sitting between two young women in hippy attire on a doorstep opposite the chapel. Interestingly, his antagonism evokes a prevailing image of southern Italy as defined by what it historically lacked in relation to an ideal model of northern Italian cities: namely, a bourgeoisie, among other factors (Gribaudi 1996). Matteo's voice is directed towards a small group, among whom I recognize the face of a university professor who is also studying the contemporary buzz around the tarantula. A debate is going on about whether anybody would still come to pay their respects to St Paul or whether all were here in vain, wishfully thinking things were still going to happen. 'Get lost! Go away!' Again and again Matteo defends this site, appropriated this year for his own needs, echoing through his own proprietary manner the middle-class bullying he is attacking, while, perhaps, distancing himself from his own – possibly middle-class – upbringing. Annalù moves over to him, conveying some restraining words in passing.

Inside the chapel, meanwhile, the altar carries the traces of other devotees. There is a bottle of milk. It was left by one devotee, a young woman in her thirties, well-known for her striking voice. There is also a piece of round bread, left by a middle-aged man, with ragged hair, torn trousers, bare feet and a strong smell of alcohol, who is now distributing pieces of another loaf to everyone present.

An elderly lady dressed all in black (perhaps an ex-tarantata?) appears on the chapel threshold. A man is by her side. Their manner radically distinguishes them from those who have come so far. The woman walks reluctantly, trailing a little behind her companion, clearly disturbed and unsettled. Is it the crowd looking on? Is it the memories this site stirs up? Is it the fear of what it might bring alive? She kneels a few steps away from the altar, keeping a little behind her companion's legs as if to shield herself, while making the sign of the cross. Her lips move in prayer.

After no more than a minute or two, both leave in restrained haste. An air of relief moves through the small room. Everyone starts to breathe again, moving joints gone stiff. For a moment, our attention had been completely captivated and I am left in awe: a split-second sense of the deep-seated, possibly apprehensive, devotion that has brought so many to this shrine, stage of the last public performances of tarantism.[7] This perception evokes images of the tarantate in my mind, footage shot by Gianfranco Mingozzi in Galatina in the early 1960s.[8]

> *A tarantata all dressed in white drags her feet to the chapel entrance, leaning heavily on two supporters. Another is carried over the threshold. Her limbs drop loosely and heavily. Inside the chapel the light is dim. Flames, brought here as signs of devotion, flicker through the red plastic of cylindrical wax containers. An old lady lies on the only available bench. Her fingers clasp the hand of a man sitting by her petrified face. A hooded figure squats on the altar step. A young girl in white kneels in front of St Paul's barricaded statue, while a relative supports her from behind. Another tarantata has climbed on top of the altar. Her head leans against St Paul's tapestry, as if listening attentively, hopefully. Voices and prayers ring through the air. They are melodic,*

desperate, grateful and occasionally punctuated by the piercing cry of the tarantate: 'A-hi!' Inquisitive faces, framed in sunlight, peer through the chapel's portal. The crowd outside is packed tightly. Some are there for the festival, many to witness the tarantate.

The mass of onlookers splits open at a tarantata's command. Dressed in black she approaches the chapel on her knees, cutting an aisle into the surrounding throng. She moves, at first, as if lame or injured. Then, suddenly, she is on her feet, galloping back and forth. The crowd retreats as her steps carve out a large circle. Her arm thrashes upwards threatening the film camera shooting from an overlooking balcony. A policeman seeks to calm her male assistant, enraged by the film crew. The afflicted continues her reckless rounds. Her guardian stands motionless, hands on hips. She begins to swirl on the spot and he moves close, holding his arms around her body and skilfully catching it as she drops backwards, unconscious, it seems. With a slight gesture he summons the policeman nearby to pass over a cushion lying ready, which he tucks under her tousled hair.

The festival procession passes [see Fig. 1.1]. Accompanied by a band, the papier mâché statue of St Paul and golden bust of St Peter are paraded through the city centre. Clergy in full ceremonial attire lead the way past gaudy market stalls and underneath arched festival frameworks of bright, coloured light bulbs.[9] A tarantata races out of the chapel attacking and splitting the crowd. A policeman blocks her attempts to reach the procession and she is taken back to the chapel with three others controlling her convulsions and resistance. More tarantate arrive. Others leave.

A tug on my arm brings me back to the present, interrupting the movie passing in my mind. Marilena Angrisani greets me. She is from Naples, in her twenties, and it is the third year we meet at Galatina. Her graduate thesis was based on a month of fieldwork on women's views of tarantism (Angrisani 2000). Like her there are others I only ever see on this occasion, once a year. Michela Almiento also completed a thesis on the tarantate (Almiento 1990). From Brindisi and now in her forties, she is one of the few to have participated in the last rituals reported to have taken place here in the late 1980s and early 1990s. Her friendship with the tarantata who danced then has brought her back each year to face St Paul together with this elderly lady. We met initially through my own research.

Then I greet Ada Metafune, physiotherapist and well-known dancer of the pizzica. We know each other well, but I have never seen her in Galatina before. She has told me how her life has been marked by the pizzica, leading her to describe herself as a modern tarantata.

We squat next to each other in the chapel, waiting, and she tells me that she has always wanted to come, but has never quite managed to make it at four in the morning. 'Perhaps I wasn't ready?' she wonders. 'But this year I told myself we're going!' She invites me to her house later in the day. A television crew has asked her to re-enact a ritual dance for them. She has done this many times, on stage and for the camera, but insists that this will be the last: 'I want to hang up the frock of the tarantate! It's as if I've passed that phase now, as if this last time today will close the circle. It's not by chance that they've asked me to do this just now.' Once again, just like Matteo's reference to the rain, coincidences are read like omens, as personal trajectories are seen to cross those of the external world in more than a random manner, creating a sense of invisible forces at play.

I meet Fabio. 'There're always lots of disrespectful people,' he says. 'Maybe this year we too can do something to maintain a bit of respect!' Clearly Annalù isn't the only one concerned about safeguarding this occasion. She knows this place and most people there. She is also the first to announce the arrival of another newcomer: 'Look who's coming! Crazy horse!' She uses the English words to refer to the nickname of this strongly built man in his early thirties: Claudio 'Cavallo' (literally meaning 'horse') Giagnotti and his group Mascarimirì are well-known for their progressive approach to Salentine popular music or 'trad-innovazione', as they like to call it (Romano 2006; Colopi and Giagnotti 2008).

It is almost 6 a.m. when a car finally stops directly in front of the chapel entrance. It is carrying a tiny elderly lady, wrapped in black and accompanied by four relatives. Like a magnet, their arrival gathers the waiting crowd dispersed in the vicinity into a tight throng around the chapel entrance. The tiny woman is Evelina. She gets out of the car without any assistance and steps towards the chapel. I haven't seen her for a while. She extends both hands to me in greeting, but keeps on walking. It is St Paul she has come to see and he is the one she must greet. A few steps into the shrine, a shrill cry emanates from her body and her arms fly up, as if hit by a laser beam radiating from the tapestry depicting St Paul above the altar. She collapses into the arms of two family members, who gently place her nimble body onto a sheet and cushion spread out on the ground. She lies there, immobile, for a few minutes. The air in the chapel is dense with anticipation. Onlookers line the walls, standing or crouching, seemingly sunk away in contemplation, with a combination of respect and curiosity creating a strange mix of outwardly attentive introspection.

After no more than a few minutes, Evelina begins to move her limbs and opens her eyes. Her daughter-in-law helps her to her feet and space is made on the small bench flanking the chapel wall, where she sits quietly, lost in herself, looking strained and extremely tired. For almost half a century now, coming to Galatina has proven to be the only balm for her suffering. 'Sometimes, in June, we had to come three or four times a day,' says her son. His wife adds: 'In 1968, it was much worse. Now for some ten years she has been better. It's strange, since there's no apparent reason. They say that when the tarantula that bites you dies you feel better too, but you mustn't take Evelina as an example. She doesn't move much and never danced.'[10]

Evelina's offering to the saint has always been that of a pilgrimage, channelling her crises according to modified ritual terms, more acceptable than ritual dances, although officially dismissed by Catholic doctrine. Traumatic events have conditioned her life: the death of her brother and father at an early age and the birth of her child out of wedlock. Condemned to remain single by social and religious mores, she has increasingly isolated herself in her homestead, with trips to work on the fields and her pilgrimage to Galatina becoming exceptional forays beyond its walls.

This year she appears to be in better shape. Often, in the past, she would faint before leaving the house on St Paul's day and her family had to drive her to Galatina unconscious. In previous years, her grandson tells, 'she was lying on the back seat, giving off muffled sounds. Her fingers were clawed together like the fangs of a spider, occasionally twitching, as if wanting to grab or bite something.'[11] The tarantula's presence is identified in Evelina's bodily state of rigidity and as a common part of her environment. 'La nonna (Gran)', as she is affectionately called, 'seems to attract spiders. In the fields too, there are always some around her. She never kills them.'[12] Even in the absence of music and dance, the feared spider is seen to have singled out Evelina.

Now too, in the chapel, she is the centre of everyone's attention, although many squat or lean against the chapel walls as if lost in prayer or contemplation, not wanting to appear too inquisitive. Suddenly, the fulcrum of attention swerves. Matteo is carried into the chapel, having abandoned himself to the arms of Fernando and

Cavallo. Evelina blurs out of focus as they place him on the ground by the altar steps. Matteo's pleas to St Paul blend with those to Cavallo: 'Aiutami! Suona per me!' (Help me! Play for me!) Cavallo stands, hands drooping indecisively by the side of his large body, uncertain, it seems, about how to react. Someone brings in a tambourine and Fernando speaks out in a firm, quiet voice: 'Can we all leave?' Evelina's son is the first to exit. Others move towards the door, hesitating at the threshold, through which the lens of a video camera cranes. Even Evelina is disturbed. She gets to her feet and, accompanied by her daughter-in-law, moves to the small room behind the altar closed off by a thick red curtain. Before leaving the chapel she must urinate (her family brings a plastic container carried in an inconspicuous paper bag) to expel what is tormenting her in a final act of release. Once again, bodily fluids cross bodily boundaries, reversing the direction of poison seen to be injected through the skin's surface. Then Evelina too leaves the chapel with the rest of her family.

I sit for a split second more, torn between the desire and curiosity to observe what will happen and the request for everyone to leave. I decide to leave and consequently rely on the fragmented tales of others to describe what happened next behind the closed chapel door, acting as both a visual and a partial acoustic barrier. Initially, I am told, a few people managed to remain in the chapel. A man came out calling for a young girl for whom Matteo had asked. Ada recounts later how Matteo furiously beat around himself at the outset and she had found herself the target of one of his blows. We joke about this (perhaps with more than an ounce of belief?), evoking contagious magic: no doubt, he will have conveyed some vital energy to her for her performance later that day. Eventually, others confirm, only Cavallo with his tambourine and the young female friend had remained in the chapel with Matteo. When he finally exited, one witness remarks later, it seemed without doubt that he had found relief.

In the meantime, I accompany Evelina and her family into the church and we move to the same row of seats as each year. At the end of the service, Evelina and her daughter-in-law go up to the altar to take communion. Then we move on, as in previous years, to the niche where the bust of St Peter stands, before circling the pews to the other side wing to see the statue of the saviour himself: St Paul. His papier mâché figure is imposingly spotlighted from below. Elevated on a pedestal above the ground, it stands among flowers and behind neat rows of electric lights, each lit by a devotee's prayer and a coin or two tinkling into the wooden box of offerings.

St Paul's robes are a striking red and green. One arm is poised across his chest, while his weight rests lightly on his left sandalled foot, accentuating the long, silver sword he is carrying like a walking stick. By his feet, on either side, two cherubs hover in space: one carries an open book, the other a green serpent stretching through the air. The apostle's gaze is framed by his bearded face and crowned by rays of gold. A number of devotees stretch across the line of lights to touch his gown, his feet, his body, securing his blessing through direct contact. Sometimes a paper handkerchief is used and then safely tucked away into a pocket or handbag. St Paul's followers are numerous and it seems that most citizens of Galatina come to see him at least once during the festival days. Others arrive from elsewhere. For many the tarantula is nowhere in the picture.

For Evelina's family, meanwhile, the spider is present and the reason behind their prayers and the lighting of yet another small lamp or more at St Paul's feet. Eventually, at a relaxed pace, we leave the church and cross the main square to the local Eros Bar for a coffee. A few sips of strong caffeine mark the end of this year's visit. Evelina's may not be a ritual of music and dance, but it is nevertheless a pilgrimage with ritualized phases: the passage to Galatina by car; a visit to the chapel of St Paul; attendance at the early morning service; a quick drink in the nearest bar; and, finally, the return journey home. As we say goodbye, a young man (years later I discover he is from Ostuni, near Brindisi, and also doing research on tarantism) approaches Evelina together with a friend, asking whether they could say goodbye to her. They shake her hand and kiss her cheeks.

Later our paths cross, and both ask, a little worried, if it had been inopportune of them to greet Evelina. It didn't seem so to me, yet, inevitably, their gesture creates a mark, an aura attributed to Evelina by way of their move, reminiscent of those seeking contact with St Paul's statue to guarantee his blessing. She is one of the very few still propelled to Galatina in the midst of crises and, as such, stands as a bridge between the tarantate of history and present circumstances in which the tarantate have gained new fame. I wonder what significance this tiny, elderly lady holds in the eyes of these two young men. I never did find out, as they leave quickly, almost timidly, but I imagine she may represent a living memorial to the rituals that once marked the territory of the Salento and are now retrospectively spectacularized (if not glorified), as well as a source of hope for those going through crises themselves.

Evelina and her family have left and I find myself jolted back to a different present. Once again my gaze extends to a wide angle, taking in what is happening all around the square. I wander across the square to a bar next to the chapel. Downstairs there is a small group of people I had met earlier: Fernando, Michela, Fabio, Enza. The conversation swerves to Matteo's case, as we struggle to confront this incident with the existing categories in our minds. Was his behaviour acceptable or completely out of place? Was it real or put on? My immediate feeling was that his behaviour was one of imitation and manipulation, highly desiring of attention. Condemning his actions, I realized I was rejecting him for precisely the reasons for which the tarantate have been accused for centuries: for putting on a show while asking for a cure – an apparent paradox that is anything but new. Already in 1771, the English traveller Burney was convinced that tarantism was 'an imposition practised by the people of Apulia to gain money: that not only the cure but the malady itself is a fraud' (Burney 1771: 313). By the year 2001, this notion of fraud or fiction has not lost its pertinence. On the contrary, it appears more acute than ever, turning a spotlight on the link between performance and therapy: is the 'show' part of the cure? Or is it the best way of avoiding the steps and changes required for recovery to take place and essentially maladaptive? My sense is that both are possible. Later in the day, watching Ada dance would allow me to reflect further on this.

In the meantime, in the Galatina bar, people's views differ. Fernando is adamant: 'Matteo is a tarantato. In my opinion, what happened today has only, once again, verified prejudices towards tarantism. The tarantate in the past, too, were 'faking', in the sense of finding an alternative route of cathartic escape, and, perhaps, also conscious of this. In the end, each one of us here is a tarantato for some reason or another.' 'What happened this morning', Enza disagrees, 'is different from what happened in the past, to the tarantate. For them, the moment of trance was important. This morning, there was none of that.' 'I wanted to throw Matteo out of the chapel,' Fabio responds vehemently:

> I felt that his behaviour was disrespectful towards the tarantate. In the
> past, they had no choice. It was the only way of getting better. It was the

only way out that peasant culture presented. But Matteo doesn't know anything about this culture. Don't get me wrong. He's a friend, I'm fond of him and I don't like to see him suffer, but I don't agree with what happened this morning. It's a personal issue. It has nothing to do with tarantism!

Relationship, work and health problems are mentioned as triggers for Matteo's presence in Galatina. Disjunctures appear to mark all major webs of his life and we may wonder to what extent his problems were also related to the fact that the display of his crisis could not be enacted in his home, in the presence of key people in his life.

A little while later, I come across Cavallo and others talking just outside the chapel. Cavallo is one of the stars of this morning's show, yet right now, clearly, this isn't a suit he is too keen to wear. 'What really bothered me', he points out, 'were all the people there. It's not like I feel at ease doing this kind of thing. There is also the woman from Scorrano who comes to ask me to play for her. But I never have. I just give her a tape.' He is referring to one of the few other elderly tarantate who apparently still performed rituals at Galatina in the 1990s. Months later, I meet Cavallo on the streets of Lecce and he mentions that, since playing for Matteo, he has gained prestige as a musician in the eyes of some. Although he himself does not seem to live this experience unambiguously, others have invested it with their own meanings: he was elected, he was seen as capable of intervening, he had, perhaps, had a glimpse of another reality, that of tarantism, glorified now that it was apparently, and with the exception of a few cases, out of reach. Crisis and celebrity seem to feed each other. Being catapulted into playing for someone in crisis has boosted Cavallo's celebrity, almost independently of his own will.

Clearly, the notion of tarantism is used to reflect many different realities. At first glance, show business, fashion and fun appear to have replaced issues of personal crisis. At the same time, they may also serve to deflect these. Beyond the open, public and academic discourses on the tarantula's dance, there are other private, more silent discourses founded largely on direct, visceral experiences of the tarantula's music and dance.

A key question that arose for me, however, on this morning of 29 June 2001, was whether Matteo and Evelina really wanted to get better. Were they ready to make the changes required to overcome what was making them suffer? Or were their actions in effect reinforcing the status quo of what was making them suffer? My feeling was that the powerful myth of the tarantula (considering particularly its revitalized fame) can and could work both ways: as a way of accessing alternative and potentially curative experiences and perspectives on reality with the assistance of others, as well as a way of demanding change from others so as not to put oneself in jeopardy of change. In this sense, 'putting on a show' may act either to confront or to conceal crises.

Dances on Screen: Invention versus Intention

The tarantate were attributed various degrees of celebrity or notoriety throughout history: they were well-known and their rituals attracted attention. The critiques of Matteo appear to mirror this historical paradox of being both revered and castigated. A look at two performances captured on film – one performed with the prime aim of healing in 1959 and the other staged for a television series in 2001 – and the contexts in which they are taken and shown reveal key issues regarding the authenticity of enactments and the centrality of intentions in the performative process.

Maria's 1959 Domestic Ritual: a Historical Performance

A small, crowded room sets the scene. It is lit up by two flickering candles and by the rays of the sun falling from a door frame and tiny window. An unmade bed leans against one wall, tipping to the ground on one side, as if two of its legs have been amputated to allow its occupant to roll effortlessly onto the floor. A small altar with religious images framed by flowers hangs from the wall and on the bedside table next to a flask of water stands a picture of St Peter and Paul. A red cloth masks the chimney, with a crucifix on its mantelpiece. The floor is cleared, except for a few chairs and benches on the edge, seating observers and the musicians, including recently deceased violinist Luigi Stifani, a guitarist and an accordion and tambourine player. A white sheet is spread across the ground, delimiting the ritual perimeter. In one corner stands a basket with offerings of money and paper icons depicting St Peter and Paul. Within the sheet's contours, a young woman lies prostrate. She must be in her late twenties. Her dress and belt are white, and her ruffled skirt reveals long, white underwear, frilled at the ends. She is barefoot and her hair falls over her face and shoulders in tousled strains. Underneath, her expression is harsh and immobile, punctuated by eyes that open and close in response to the pizzica beats reverberating through the room.

These are images of the dance of Maria of Nardò, rendered famous among the tarantate by Ernesto De Martino's book *La terra del rimorso* (1961a), the most in-depth and well-known study on tarantism to date. The film *La terapia coreutico-musicale del tarantismo* (Carpitella 1960) shows her dance on 24 June 1959 (De Martino 2005: 38–46), and is, to my knowledge, the first cinematographic document of these rituals, despite the many mutations already affecting this tradition as socio-economic and religious pressures were leading to its demise. Maria's dance, as captured in Carpitella's film, is one of the only domestic rituals not staged for the camera documented on celluloid. Ever since, with a few exceptions, photographers and camera teams have had to rely on reproductions: staged rituals performed by tarantate, or substitute actors, paid to do so.[13]

Forty-two years later, for the festival of St Peter and Paul on 30 June 2001, this original footage is projected onto a massive screen hoisted in front of the baroque façade of Galatina's main church on the San Pietro piazza. A spotlighted stage flanks the canvas sheet across which black and white figures move: shots of Maria's ritual and others of the tarantate performing their crises on the very pavement now packed with the film's standing audience. A strange disjuncture appears: moments of the past, hovering ghostlike a few metres above the ground, continuing to place a spell on those looking on, now safe to wear whatever colour they please, with a remote-control option to switch off a performance that the Church fought to extinguish for centuries. It is a screened, carefully canned version of tarantism, available in easily digestible portions, and subsequently washed (and danced) down to the beat of the pizzica and other Salentine music, as various local bands perform on stage [see Fig. 8.1]. Meanwhile, the ritual filmed by Carpitella (1960) continues on screen, and I elaborate it here with details from De Martino's (De Martino 2005: 38–44) written accounts of the very same ritual:

Four men in light summer clothes and sandals play the violin, tambourine, guitar and accordion. Their faces are marked by fatigue, the effect of playing from dawn to dusk, with nothing but brief breaks. Their notes bombard the distraught-looking woman lying lethargically on the floor without reacting to the melodies proposed. Then, triggered by a new piece, she begins to move, taking up the rhythm. Her feet tap and her head moves rapidly from side to side. *She shuffles across the floor on her shoulders, increasing the momentum. Knees arched, she propels herself backwards on alternate heels, circling the entire ritual perimeter with her arms stretched out or folded on her chest. At one point, she tries to thread her body through the legs of a wicker chair, which tumbles over.*[14] *She follows, rolling over and over, moving across the floor. She wrenches herself forward on her stomach, seeking the proximity of the instruments, as if hungry to absorb, almost touch, every note.*

The violinist kneels down in response to her approach. His bow moves close to her ear and propels her onto her knees with her hands crouched in front of her, chest tipping rhythmically from side to side, embodying mutual interactions of 'call and response'.[15] *Abruptly, the tarantata springs to her feet and runs in circles, never losing the rhythm. Her moves include those of the pizzica, some danced on the spot, while a handkerchief, clasped between both hands, marks others. Her feet hit the ground rapidly, over and over again: stamping, crushing, destroying.*

Without warning a newcomer appears at the door, dressed in a bright red and yellow striped pullover. The young tarantata becomes agitated and wavers visibly. The intruder is chased away with violent accusations, but the invisible chord between dancer and musicians has snapped. The tarantata remains perturbed, as if inebriated and fails to respond to the rhythm the musicians strike up again. Quickly, coloured ribbons are sought in remedy, as colours, like sounds and movements, are part of the ritual remedy kit. Different ribbons are thrown towards the young woman. She ignores them at first. Then a red one provokes her attention. She grabs the strip of fabric, fixes it with her gaze and shreds it to pieces with her teeth. Only then does she gradually pick up the musical rhythm again and the ritual framework is retrieved.

Eventually the rounds danced by the young tarantata diminish in circumference. She twirls in a pirouette, loses the rhythm and collapses. Prepared arms bolster her fall and gently lower her head onto a cushion. A cover is draped over her resting limbs. The musicians stop playing and wipe off their sweat. Water and food are brought for refreshment, but the pause is only brief. The dance must go on. Only late in the evening does the music stop as a man bursts into the house, angrily dispelling the crowd. He is the employer of the young dancer and urgently anticipates her return to work. It is he who has anticipated the money (to be worked off by the tarantata later on) to pay the musicians. For the time being, treatment is rescheduled for the following day.

The next morning, the first musical chords stretch the tarantata's body into an arc: her spine flexes into a bridge resting on her strained neck and heels.[16] *Within a few seconds she drops onto her back and rolls off the bed onto the ground. Numerous dance cycles are repeated. A short break is taken at noon, and only in the early afternoon, winks between experienced bystanders confirm the first signs that recovery is close. The afflicted had eaten a little earlier. She keeps on emitting short, shrill screams. Her dance phases are shorter now and show a greater variety of steps. Then, finally, she breaks off in mid-cycle, signals to the musicians to stop playing and steadfastly walks to her bed. Relief spreads through the room. Just to be sure this is for real a last tune is played. It is dedicated to St Paul. The young tarantata remains insensitive to the music and, grateful for her recovery, everyone present kneels in prayer. Later that day she dances once more at Galatina, in the chapel of St Paul. It was he, she confirms, who has saved her yet again, whispering in dialect into her ears: 'I grant you grace.'*

The life of the tarantata Maria, as recounted by De Martino (2005: 38–46), is marked early by the spider's bite: her father dies when she is young; at eighteen she falls in love with a man whose family disapproves of her and, rejected in this way, she first succumbs to the tarantula. She is compelled to dance and eventually persuaded, in spite of St Paul's demands to join her in mystical union, to marry another man who is often ill and out of work. Nevertheless, St Paul rules as her spiritual spouse and her annual afflictions allow her to participate in the celebrations of his feast day. At the time of writing, I am told, Maria continues to pay her respects at Galatina.[17]

Ada's 2001 Dance on TV: a Contemporary Performance

In the afternoon of 29 June 2001, as I drive to see Ada, I have no doubts that her performance for the cameras of the Canale 5 television crew will merely reinforce the gaping chasm widely perceived between past and present spider dances. However, this prognosis also turns out to be too simplistic.

At Ada's house, in the south-west Salento, the film crew, musicians and family members are ready to set off when I arrive. In the car, Ada begins to talk:

You can't imagine how much I dreamt this afternoon. This morning I was quite well after coming back from Galatina, but sleeping now after lunch, I went through lots of things. I discharged myself with my dreams. I dreamt of a dead person, Amadeo De Rosa. He died two years ago and every year we organize a series of musical events in his memory. It was he who inspired us young people to start with the pizzica. He was there. And then I dreamt that I was dancing the pizzica and being lifted off the ground. I was literally floating. It might be significant, now that I have to dance.[18]

Once again, a fine thread of meaning is evoked to link experiences and events. This occasion is not new to Ada. She has performed the tarantate's dance often, but it is the first time she is dancing with the intention of having a final go. This date represents a symbolic stepping stone, a desired turn in a dramatic vein of events and experiences running through her adult life, surfacing soon after her marriage and the birth of her first child, and often leaving her abandoned to crises. Now she is in her early forties, the mother of two children, a physiotherapist and fitness trainer by profession and, through an association founded with her husband, engaged in promoting cultural events in her hometown. She is a radiant woman, with striking black hair and delicate facial features. Learning to dance the pizzica, she stresses, has changed her life in many ways. Above all, it has allowed her to connect with her emotions and sensuality. This, she emphasizes, is why she sees herself as a modern tarantata. In subtle interpretative stitches, she has woven the costume of the tarantate into the fabric of her personal life, connecting her own story with the precedent of other women in crisis in the region in which she was born, a precedent made accessible not only through the stories she has grown up with and sought out from elderly generations, but also through the documentaries and numerous publications booming in parallel to the tarantula's music and dance in recent years.[19]

Another car has joined us and we come to a halt on the top of a ridge that drops down to the Ionian coast, providing a splendid view of the port of Gallipoli and the surrounding coastline. The late afternoon countryside stretching to the sea is a hazy olive-silver. A few steps below the natural granite terraces where the cars are parked, there is a small church set into the rock: a cave furnished with pews, an altar and a cross at the entrance. Ironically, like the tarantate, Ada was to perform near a chapel. The filmset is prepared. Microphones and light exposures are tested, while Ada changes into a long white gown with frilled cotton trousers and touches up her make-up. Barbara, a young woman and passionate dancer from her hometown, gives her a hand and then hugs her tightly, noticing how emotional she has become. Ada's eyes are filled to the brim. She comes up to me, saying: 'Dammi un bacio' (Give me a kiss), acknowledging what was going on inside her, making Barbara and me aware of this intimate space, somehow pulling us in.

The musicians begin to warm up. There are five of them now, with four tambourines and an accordion. They are all men, members of various local music groups. None of them is specifically dressed for the occasion, their sandals, cotton trousers and T-shirts being their usual summer attire. Ada and her mother, petite in a flowery dress, prepare the ritual space on an even stone surface. They remove small pebbles and twigs and then unfold a large white sheet, with a lace edge, over a slight padding of mats taken from the cars around. The sheet is spread with ritual objects, reminders of tarantism's syncretism with Catholicism, while at the same time, perhaps, mirroring Ada's individual preferences: an image of St Paul, coloured ribbons, a red scarf, a string of bells. Then all is set.

Ada's expression is one of concentration and anguish. She stands a few metres from the ritual sheet, in between her mother and Barbara, now dressed all in black for the occasion, one arm hooked into each of theirs. The music starts. Slowly, extremely slowly, the group of three women moves towards the ritual space. Ada's soles drag heavily across the ground and her head tips to one side as she abandons herself to the performance. The musicians play in line, with their backs to the magnificent coastal setting. Their manner appears automatic, detached. Ada collapses onto the sheet, still supported by her two female assistants. She lies face down on the ground, hardly moving at first. A mop of hair hides her face. Close up, through my own camera lens, the scene is a colour version of black and white photos of Maria of Nardò's dance. Slowly, she begins to stir in heavy, listless motions. Then her rhythm picks up, she rolls over and over, gets to her feet, moves close to the musicians with her head between her hands and two tambourines, dances and then collapses onto the hard ground. Her mother remains close by at all times, occasionally adjusting the sheet as it shrivels up and out of place.

Two cameras move around Ada, in between her and the musicians, like hungry mouths and overextended gazes, lustful where she is listless. Never, however, is she interrupted or told what to do. No more than fifteen minutes pass in all. In between, I have my own (camera) crisis, perhaps indicative of my own degree of participation: in a hectic attempt to replace my used-up film, I open the camera without rewinding the completed roll, tearing out the ribbon of ruined pictures as a last resort to capture at least some images of the final part of the performance. Various others are standing and sitting around the scene. Three women on a late afternoon stroll up the hill have moved close to watch. Then the music stops.

Ada sits up. She has an air of immense vulnerability, of gaping emptiness about her. Everyone tends to themselves, their instruments, the cameras, and Ada is left to her own resources without any notes or the attentive camera gaze to sustain her. Barbara zooms in to embrace her. Ada stretches to wrap her arms around the younger woman, as if clasping on to a life-belt, something to support her as she resurfaces, as she comes out of her role to face reality beyond the performance. Finally, after a few moments, she gets to her feet slowly and then moves around kissing everyone present in turn, musicians and attendants, thanking each one.[20]

Just a few minutes later, Ada is back in front of the camera, under a tree close to the cave, for an interview of some twenty minutes. When everything is finally packed up to go, the camera team from Canale 5 appears content. They are making a series, entitled 'Gentes', on popular traditions of Italy and Europe, which is to be screened nationwide in autumn 2001. Ada jokes light-heartedly in the car, telling how she had been asked to end the interview with a warning: 'State attenti alla tarantola!' (Beware of the tarantula!)

Driving back to Lecce that night, I am struck by the strong emotions Ada's performance evoked not only in her but also in me, seeing that I knew some of her story. One of the musicians I talked to at a later stage, meanwhile, remarked how disappointed he had been by the whole event, as it was too staged, too artificial. Once again the fine link between invention and intention surfaces, suggesting that faking or acting-as-if, so easily dismissed as fraud, may (or may not) have a pertinent influence on everyday reality. Ada used the setting invented for the TV crew with the intention of fulfilling her personal objective of closing a phase in her own life. Few others knew. Yet the cameras documented this moment, eventually letting the whole nation witness it. Ada's motivation was deeply meaningful on a personal level, independently of what it might mean or how it might appear to others. Her engagement went beyond that of putting on a show for Canale 5, making it both staged and not-staged at the same time.

Meanwhile, the events and discussions of 29 June 2001 left me feeling as if I'd been around an inter-looping highway system of tarantula tracks, on which Evelina's, Matteo's and Ada's crises intersected. The life stories and pilgrimages of three generations criss-crossed at Galatina, in one tiny chapel with a crumbling altar, together with those of many others who, like me, found themselves witnessing and participating with strong sentiments and animated discussions. The double-sided link between crises and celebrity emerged. Depending on the intention behind any performance, it may encompass both the curative support of others, who acknowledge the reality of issues and experiences faced by the afflicted individual, and the manipulative potential of exploiting others' attention to perpetuate and reinforce situations of affliction. The next chapter's look at the tarantula's appeal throughout history provides further evidence.

Notes

1. 'Santu Paulu meu de le tarante, pizziche le caruse tutte quante, Santu Paulu meu de Galatina, famme na grazia a mie e a tutte quante.' This is one of the most popular songs in the repertoire of Salentine musicians today.

2. The Italian words Evelina and her family use are *i guai* (literally translated as 'the troubles' or 'the difficulties').

3. Giancarlo Vallone (2004) quotes Congedo (1903) to suggest that the healing qualities of this well may be ascribed to healing spit, *lo sputo risanatore*, and that the owners of the house where St Peter and Paul apparently resided in Galatina were said to cure poisonous bites with their spit. Such treatments of poisonous bites with spit were also applied by the *sanpaolari* and others (see Chapter 6, 'Tarantula Alternatives: Choosing Treatment Options'). These references to the use of liquids in healing practices may also be linked to the relevance of rain, urine and poisons in case studies of tarantism, as well as discussions on 'fluids of healing' in medical anthropology more generally. See Hsu and Low (2007).

4. This was the entrance to the eatery Il Covo della Taranta, the den or lair of the tarantula, in the first years of the new millennium and a clothes shop for children by 2007.

5. Galatina, 29 June 1997.

6. Marina Roseman (2002: 122) points out how 'shimmering things, combining movement and light, exist at the fuzzy boundary between the visual and the kinetic, disassembling distinct sensory fields,' and thereby play a key role in bringing about experiences entangling 'the empirically observable with the magically real in a world of temporal, sensorial and experiential overlap'.

7. See Nocera (1994: 178–86) and Almiento (1994: 255–66). These accounts of rituals performed in the chapel of St Paul at Galatina in the 1990s are variously disputed or confirmed.

8. What follows is a description of snapshots from this footage.

9. Salentine festivals are characterized by elaborate street illuminations composed of coloured light-bulb designs, known as *luminarie*, creating a festive atmosphere and leaving streets bright as daylight even at night-time.

10. Galatina, 29 June 1997. Evelina's relation to the tarantula is mediated by the figure of St Paul and her pilgrimage in his honour rather than music or dance. Nevertheless, I present her situation here, as she is the only tarantata who still openly manifests her affliction at Galatina. Moreover, her annual pilgrimage constitutes a performative event shaping her story and is indicative of a larger context of entanglements within which the tarantula is seen to intervene.

11. Galatina, 29 June 1997.

12. Ibid.

13. It remains unclear as to what the earliest audio-visual registrations of tarantism are. In 1959, De Martino and his team took photos, as well as film and sound recordings of the tarantate in the Salento. Franco Pinna's photographs have been published in Pinna (2002) and in *La terra del rimorso* (De Martino 1961a), the first edition of which was accompanied by a registration of recordings made inside the chapel of St Paul in Galatina. Diego Carpitella's footage was reproduced in the documentary *La terapia coreutico-musicale del tarantismo* (1960). This was later included in Gianfranco Mingozzi's film *Sulla terra del rimorso* (1982), which was reproduced in video format in 2002 and in DVD format in 2007 (Nardò: Besa) and sold together with the book *La taranta* (Mingozzi 2002), containing the complete film script. Other pictures by photographers Franco Pinna, Arturo Zavattini and Ando Gilardi appear in the book *I viaggi nel Sud di Ernesto De Martino* (Gallini and Faeta 1999). Earlier sound recordings were registered by Alan Lomax and Diego Carpitella in 1954 (Brunetto 1995: 139–47), and reproduced on the CD *Italian Treasury: Puglia: The Salento*, edited by Goffredo Plastino (2002, Alan Lomax Collection). For further musical sources, see also Agamennone (2005), Attanasi (2007) and Chiriatti et al. (2007).
14. The tarantate were said to weave themselves through chairs in imitation of the spider weaving its web.
15. These interactions bring to mind relationships between dancers and musicians in many West African and sub-Saharan African musical traditions (Chernoff 1979), as well as those described by Deidre Sklar (2001) in her account of dance performances during festivities in honour of the Virgin of Guadaloupe.
16. The tarantate were typically said to perform this movement, also described as a 'hysteric arc'.
17. Maurizio Nocera, 1 April 2006, referring to June 2005.
18. Interestingly, Ada's dream relates to descriptions of trance dancing elsewhere, such as among the Temiar of Malaysia: trance dancers speak of 'soaring above the forest canopy and circling the mountain tops' (Roseman 1993: 162) while dancing.
19. Various publishers – Aramirè, Besa, Capone, to name just a few – specialize in publications regarding the tarantula's music and dance.
20. This tender moment of 'resurfacing' is described in connection with trance dances elsewhere. Edward Schieffelin (1996: 77) speaks of how, 'coughing and gasping', a Kaluli medium in Papua New Guinea 'returned to the living'. Roseman (1993: 162) tells of how other participants help Malaysian Temiar dancers who have fainted back onto their feet, and by 'supporting them around the waist ... begin to dance them back to consciousness', to their 'true heart' and 'true eyes', thereby choreographing 'themes of community support and interdependence' (ibid.: 165).

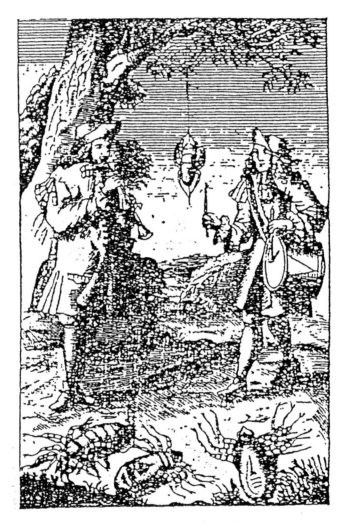

Fig. 2.1 From *Observations Rares de Médecine*, 1758
(reprinted in Scholes 1964). This work asserts that the
insects will dance rhythmically if a tarantella tune is
played to them (source: Oxford University Press).

Chapter 2
Webs through Time:
Origins and History of Tarantism

The symbol of the taranta
lends a figure to the formless,
rhythm and melody to menacing silence,
and colour to the colourless ...
The symbol offers a perspective
for imagining, hearing and watching
what we lack imagination for
and are deaf and blind to,
and which nevertheless peremptorily
asks to be imagined, heard and seen.

De Martino 2005: 36

Once upon a time, Satan compelled a malicious woman to harm the Virgin Mary of Finisterrae. This woman captured a number of tarantulas and, knowing they were poisonous, placed them in the alms caskets of the Madonna's church. Henceforth, all who came to leave a coin or two in devotion were treacherously bitten in their hands. Fear and anguish spread among the faithful and, suspecting witchcraft, many began to abandon the Madonna's shrine. The Virgin Mary, in turn, spoke to the spiders: 'You were born without malice, but an evil woman taught you to act in an immoral way. Now you will do the same for punishment and everyone will be afraid of you. No longer will you be spiders bringing gain. Instead, you will bring death.' By virtue of her powers, the Virgin directed the rays of the ferocious July sun onto the tarantulas and the atrocious heat drove them to madness. They poisoned each other, contorted themselves in agony, fled into the woods and then took revenge against the evil woman by developing a preference to bite women. Through their poisonous bite they transferred their own misfortune, the agony of convulsions and madness, onto their victims.

Thus goes the legend of Sanarica, a small town not far from Santa Maria di Leuca on the southernmost tip of the Salento, also known as Finisterrae: end of the earth (Bronzini 1976: 136). This story places Satan at the origins of tarantism. One woman falls for his powers and the tarantula spiders become her tool. One curse is offset by another and the spiders, ever since, dance to the Madonna's tune. The tarantulas are depicted as no more than playing cards in a classic match of good against evil. They are props for the two-sided roles of tyrants and victims, symbolically imbued with the power of whomever they come to represent. They are cards in the hands of others, and yet with a sting (and valency) of their own, played out in reaction to an original sin, the original pact with Satan on which their own doom depends: the original sin of a woman, for which all other women must pay. Christian imagery is blatant in this game, reminiscent of another downfall and another temptation, represented by the powerful symbols of an apple and a snake. The legend of Finisterrae wraps tarantism into Christian mythology. Its roots are equated with Satan. The tarantate seem to be placed into Eve's shoes and, in this way, a complex ritual – with probable pagan foundations – is cut and filed to fit any golden frame on a Christian church wall.

A look at the possible origins and the widely documented histories of tarantism provides a perfect illustration of how understandings of cause and effect in the context of affliction and cure, as well as forms of intervention considered appropriate, are inevitably located historically and culturally. 'By writing on tarantism,' writes Martha Baldwin (1997: 185), 'the physician could advocate his own philosophical allegiance and demonstrate its ability to account for new medical phenomena. Rather than being concerned with treating ailing patients, the early modern physician was eager instead to explain the forces of nature at work in the world.' Tarantism has been (and continues to be) decoded in numerous ways. What seventeenth-century Apulians consider a radical treatment against the tarantula's poison was dispelled as deception by an English traveller of the same era (Burney 1771). What a twenty-first-century woman may live as a turning point in her life is presented on television to the rest of her nation as the spectacularized reproduction of a long-dead ritual tradition. A link to the tarantula spider, continuously reweaving its own interpretative web, appears to be the only constant fixture in this game. A look back in time reveals diverse explanations of tarantism and, most of all, the historical specificity of each. Moreover, the often indistinguishable real and invented past inevitably colours the present. In the modern Salento, views about how things are believed to have been are flashed as trump cards of how things should, ideally, be.

Possible Origins: Searching for Tarantism's Roots

The precise roots of tarantism remain a mystery. A 1426 document written by the Venetian doctor Sante Ardoini, and printed in the *Sertum papale de venenis* series, is most commonly cited as the first literary evidence of tarantism. This text describes the spider's victims as subject to a severe state of melancholy and a compulsive impulse to dance. It also refers to earlier texts that mention afflictions by the tarantula in the Mediterranean area without, however, making any reference to music or dance. Goffredo Malaterra (1724), for instance, tells how Norman soldiers bitten by spiders during the 1043 siege of Palermo were treated with hot compresses.[1] George Mora (1963: 419) challenged the historical primacy of Ardoini's account, arguing that a 1362 edition of the same *De venenis* series, attributed to Guglielmo De Marra, constitutes 'the oldest document dealing with the musical exorcism of people supposedly bitten by the tarantula ... The concept is expressed in it – somewhat obscurely – that the *melodic bite of the arachnoid* makes possible the re-evocation of the bite in musical terms' (Thorndike 1934: 526–34). Gabriele Mina's (2000) extensive research has since confirmed this.

The origins of tarantism have been sought in different times and places. Ernesto De Martino (2005: 215) relegates the emergence of this ritual practice to the period between the ninth and fourteenth centuries, drawing on historical evidence to show how tarantism developed out of a continuum of adaptations required for survival. The actual danger of spider poisoning was widely reported in Apulia. At the same time, its shores were not only subject to Islamic invasions, but also a stopover point for the crusaders on their way to the Holy Land.

The designated period up to the fourteenth century marks the time span from the height of Islam's expansion to the Occident's eventual counter-reaction. According to De Martino, tarantism arose out of the dual need to deal with actual spider epidemics and changing socio-political and religious conditions. The experience of spider poisoning provided a model to deal with social crises, such as those arising out of religious conflicts plaguing Apulia, as the symptoms of the tarantate closely resembled those of actual spider bites.

Despite the obscure origins of tarantism, the mythic tarantula itself had actual, zoological ancestors, notwithstanding disputes about which spider type was to blame. Although this explanation does not provide any indication as to why music rather than any other treatment was used, this link to a naturalistic cause, supported by a vast collection of medical literature, is likely to be one reason why tarantism has persisted into the present century despite the Church's persecution of non-Christian beliefs (Sigerist 1948: 112–14; Rouget 1986: 162; Bartholomew 1994: 288; Di Mitri 1995: 226). Ethnomusicologist Gilbert Rouget (1986: 162), defining tarantism in terms of possession, supports this point:

> The Church of Rome could never for a moment have tolerated its existence as an overt possession cult. The bite of the tarantula, whose effects coincide so extraordinarily closely with the signs that herald the onset of possession, provided a providential alibi ... Women who gave themselves up to these practices were no longer sinners but unfortunate victims of the tarantula.

Other precedents of tarantism have been sought in the European dancing manias, St Vitus's or St John's dance, widespread in Germany and the Netherlands in the thirteenth and fourteenth centuries (Hecker 1865: 143–91). Like tarantism, these manias appeared to be seasonally determined; they found their victims among all kinds of social and professional classes, and involved a strong aversion to certain colours, especially red. However, this link is placed in jeopardy by the fact that no mention whatsoever is made of a poisonous bite or spider. There are few documents available about the music used, but its application appears to have varied considerably from that of tarantism: St Vitus's or St John's dancers are, for instance, described as having been at the mercy of their convulsions independently of music.[2]

58

Meanwhile, more ancient parallels to tarantism have been drawn with the Dionysian, Corybante and Orphic cults of Greek origin, all of which were characterized by the cathartic use of dance and music (De Martino 1961a; Salvatore 1989; Lapassade 1994; Di Mitri 1996).[3] The fact that Apulia was part of the Magna Graecia in the fifth and fourth centuries BC and so heavily exposed to Greek influence is drawn upon as evidence. This period, however, is extremely remote in time, even if we locate the first records of tarantism in the ninth century CE as De Martino suggests. Marius Schneider (1948) retreats even further back in history to propose that tarantism has its origins in the medicinal rites of megalithic civilizations. Along similar but bolder lines, Rosario Jurlaro (1980) roots the tarantula's ritual in ancient propitiatory rites. Dancers, he proposes, mimed the wild reactions of animals bitten by a horsefly and music was used to replace the horsefly's buzzing drone.

With all these varying explanations it is valuable to remember, as historian Peregrine Horden (2000) cautions in his study on music and medicine, that the notion of continuity is always highly seductive.[4] It may conceal a variety of diverse phenomena, whose apparent continuity may well be the result of numerous small discontinuities. 'Rather than search the mists of time, we should reckon with the possibility that new healing cults, tarantism included, can develop quickly; unconnected elements can quite suddenly coalesce' (ibid:. 253). Unrelated elements may spontaneously combine to create cults or consolidate traditions, which are then – for a variety of contemporary purposes – retrospectively linked to preceding ones on the basis of common characteristics. The same reservations were expressed by the eighteenth-century traveller Henry Swinburne, who suggested that an accident may well have led to the 'discovery' of the tarantula's bite for the purposes of tarantism rituals (1783: 393).

The above qualms apply equally to ideas locating the origins of tarantism in the Salento itself. Proof for these claims is generally based on archaeological findings of recent decades, including the 1970 discovery of Palaeolithic cave paintings in the Grotta dei Cervi of Porto Badisco, near Otranto (Graziosi 1996). This find gave rise to hypotheses that initiation practices of early pagan cults were held here and diverse rock paintings are seen to be linked to the symbolism of tarantism (Tolledi 1998: 8). This applies specifically to one anthropomorphic figure known as il *dio che danza* (the dancing god) or *lo stregone danzante* (the dancing wizard). Other, more abstract designs were identified, in similar vein, as spider webs or tambourines (Giannuzzi 1996). It remains impossible to draw precise conclusions about the connection between these cave paintings and tarantism, and, although I would be careful about accepting these links, it does appear significant that, unblemished by this fact, the dancing god – just like the tarantula spider – has become a blockbuster icon in the contemporary world of the tarantula's music and dance [see Figs 7.1 and 7.2].

Etymological considerations provide other clues about the beginnings of tarantism. Most commonly the term 'tarantism' is linked to the town of Taranto, tucked into the Gulf of Taranto in the Ionian Sea (Basile 2000). To the Greeks, this ancient city was known as Taras or Tarassos and, later, under the Romans, it was called Tarentum. Its link to tarantism may be explained on the basis of the widespread existence of the tarantula spider in this area, partly due to its climatic conditions and non-intensive agriculture (Naselli 1951: 225; De Martino 2005: 213). Others argue that this link is based on the importance of Taranto in Greek and Roman times, which encouraged those who were ill to converge here to seek medical help (Baglivi 1696; De Raho 1908: 3). According to alternative opinions, the name of Taranto forms the base of the term tarantism and is associated with the Greek word for agitation, *tarassia* (Jurlaro 1980: 57). Yet others see a connection between the term tarantism and the word *terrantola*, referring to creatures living in and off the ground (Hecker 1865: 165; Katner 1956: 12).

Finally, legends, such as the story from Sanarica, posit potential explanations for the origins of tarantism. Greek mythology is also a frequently cited source. The tarantate are seen to 'unwittingly reincarnate the pursued heroines of Greek stories: Io, the woman-cow, pursued by the divine bite of Hera's horsefly; Phaedra stung by love; Arachne driven to suicide by Athena, her rival in weaving; Erigone, Icarus's daughter, who hanged herself from a tree, setting off an epidemic of hangings among young girls' (Cixous and Clément 1986: 20). Arachne's is perhaps the most frequently quoted story, although music and dance do not feature in this account.[5] One version tells how the young Arachne had embroidered an enormous tapestry depicting the stories of the gods. She displayed this work in public and, receiving numerous compliments, became guilty of arrogance and presumption. When Athena heard this, she went to see for herself and, struck with rage, tore the work to pieces. Arachne escaped to the forest, but Athena followed and found her suspended from a rope, dead. Athena brought Arachne's body back to life, transformed into that of a spider, which immediately began to weave its web. 'Weave, little one,' Athena sighed, 'from now on you will do this for a living, without glory. No longer will you be able to boast and defy the gods.'

Historical Interpretations: Explaining the Tarantula's Cult

Over the centuries, tarantism has gripped the imagination of scholars throughout Europe, some informed by the tales and accounts of others, some adventurous enough to go and see for themselves. Two key points of view fired a fierce debate about the actual or mythical character of the tarantula's bite: one musical (considering the effects of music on the human organism) and one medical (focused on the character and causes of the symptoms involved).[6] The Jesuit priest Athanasius Kircher (1641, 1673) was one of the main proponents of the musical perspective of the seventeenth-century Renaissance and humanist periods. His writings, based on the accounts of two informant priests from Lecce and Taranto, documented popular beliefs on tarantism, magic, magnetism and the therapeutic powers of music. His interpretation revived classical ideas on the correspondence between bodily humours, states of health and illness, and musical melodies seen to influence these.

Epifanio Ferdinando (1621) and Giorgio Baglivi (1696), meanwhile, were key advocates of a medical explanation of tarantism. Their ideas were based on naturalistic and positivist foundations, reducing tarantism to a medical condition of two types: a biological reaction to a toxic bite or a psychological disorder. Ferdinando, a native of the Salento familiar with cases of tarantism, dispelled explanations of the magical powers of music and, taking a physiological approach, argued instead that music facilitated dancing and perspiration, thereby expelling toxins via the skin's surface (Portulano Scoditti 1999). Baglivi, a university professor in Rome who received his information from his adoptive father in Lecce, meanwhile, concentrated on the fact

61

that many tarantate were never actually bitten by a real spider. He coined the term *carnevaletti delle donne* (women's small carnivals) to describe those who simulated the symptoms of the tarantula's bite in order to let their hair down and celebrate. Such a view of tarantism emerged from many pre-nineteenth-century English texts (Burney 1771; Turnbull 1771; Swinburne 1783) and was voiced again on 29 June 2001 as a reaction to Matteo's dance in Galatina.[7]

This confrontation between musical and medical views was catalysed by related debates in the fields of magic and science (Tomlinson 1994; Di Mitri 2006). In the eighteenth century, this conflict became particularly evident when tarantism received two blows leading to its gradual disintegration: one came with the advent of the Enlightenment, the other from the Catholic Church. The Neapolitan medical school institutionalized Cartesian scepticism, and tarantism was increasingly discounted as a mere superstition and the tarantate viewed as psychologically disturbed individuals, as the work of Francesco Serao (1742) revealed. He was a physician from Naples, with personal experiences of tarantism and extensive correspondence on this subject with Apulian informants, viewing tarantism both as a form of corruption characterizing Apulia's lower classes and as a pathological condition. Its cause, he argued, was not to be found in the tarantula spider, but rather in the melancholic disposition of Apulia's inhabitants themselves.

Catholicism brought a second blow. Attempts to control the non-Christian ritual of tarantism were best demonstrated by the coercion of mythical and biblical symbolism, as the image of the tarantula became conflated with that of St Paul. In the years following the construction of St Paul's chapel in the mid-eighteenth century in Galatina, ecclesiastical authorities played a major role in driving tarantism indoors and underground.

Meanwhile, in the eighteenth century, conflicts continued between the popular myth of the tarantula and more scientifically founded interpretations of tarantism (Convegno 1999). The ideas of the Neapolitan medical school were criticized and developed by various scholars, increasingly recognizing the cultural character of the tarantula's bite (Valetta 1706; Caputo 1741; Cirillo 1771). Nevertheless, resistance to these views persisted into the nineteenth century. It was Giuseppe Chiaia (1887) who most openly expressed a strongly anticlerical stance, seeking to prove the validity of popular beliefs on tarantism by reviving Kircher's ideas. At the same time, nineteenth- and early twentieth-century medical literature staunchly continued to reduce tarantism to spider poisoning or psychological illness (Carusi 1848; De Masi 1874; Campelli 1878; Kobert 1901). A detailed survey by Apulian doctor Francesco De Raho (1908) followed this line of enquiry. With reference to experiments on guinea pigs, De Raho concluded that the spider bite alone was not sufficient to cause the violent symptoms observed in the tarantate. Instead, he diagnosed a minor form of hysteria.

The twentieth century brought a gradual awareness of the cul-de-sac medical research had run into by ignoring the cultural aspects of tarantism. Henry Sigerist (1948), a Swiss-born doctor and one of the 'fathers of modern medical history' (Horden 2000: 22), established tarantism as a neurosis peculiar to Apulia, derived from ancient orgiastic cults and camouflaged as an illness so as to escape the Church's condemnation. Marius Schneider (1948) presented an in-depth symbolic analysis of tarantism as a seasonal and medicinal rite, expressing the cosmological understanding of megalithic peoples. His approach was based on a 'system of mystical correspondences between nature and man, between the elements, astrological signs, the seasons and sounds' (Rouget 1986: 159). Nevertheless, medical assumptions also proved to be resilient. Backman (1952) described dance epidemics such as tarantism as the result of ergot poisoning from grain and bread. Wilhelm Katner (1956) identified sunstroke as the actual pathogenic stimulus, whereas Giordano (1957) applied the category of collective psychosis to the tarantate's affliction.

Only the surface of almost a millennium of studies on tarantism can be touched on here. This vast and rich literature shows how views on tarantism have been subject to continual negotiation. The therapeutic options available to the tarantate directly related to accepted views of this ritual tradition. Its interpretations embodied not only a desire to make sense of the human condition but also an implicit play of power. Cases of tarantism threatened the influence of Christianity and the development of medical science and, as such, both institutions sought to control it through redefinition. Perhaps not surprisingly, with the turn to the twenty-first century the story of tarantism is being rewritten once again (with more or less success) as more than an antidote to fears of the millennium bug. It serves new purposes for which the flourishing market of recent editions and translations of historical texts on tarantism caters in grand style

(Mina and Torsello 2006). Among these Dorothy Zinn's English translation of De Martino's monumental work is one of the more recent (2005).

De Martino's View: a Key Point of Reference

'Have you read De Martino? Have you studied his book *La terra del rimorso*?' More often than not, this was the first question people in the Salento asked when I talked about my research. The word 'tarantism' seems to trigger, first and foremost, the name of this well-known Italian scholar and the title of his famous publication defining the tarantate's ritual as a form of musical, choreographic and chromatic exorcism. It is as if tarantism, now apparently long extinct, continues to exist on almost four hundred pages, densely packed with a rich description and interpretation of this healing ritual. For an anthropologist looking for personal stories and first-hand experiences, it becomes a frustrating white screen on which shadows dance, as paraphrased and often reductive versions of De Martino's black and white script dominate popular views of the tarantula's dance. It is impossible to consider tarantism today without taking note of this important study, suggestive of the influence of anthropological work on other contemporary movements (such as the writing of Mircea Eliade, Michael Harner and Carlos Castaneda on 'Neo-shamanism'), or the historical documentation of tarantism rituals in Spain and the United States subsequent to the translation of a book on this subject by Giorgio Baglivi (Horden 2003: 193).

In the summer months of 1959, Ernesto De Martino and his team of researchers undertook the first in-depth field study of tarantism.[8] Their research involved detailed interviews with twenty-one tarantate: sixteen women and five men between the ages of thirteen and seventy-six. The team observed both domestic dance rituals and pilgrimages to the chapel of St Paul in Galatina. Although the duration of this fieldwork did not exceed three weeks (20 June – 10 July), De Martino was able to build on contacts established in the early post-war period when he was posted to Bari and Lecce as commissioner of the Socialist Federation (Panico 1983: 140).

De Martino uncovered the power relations within which tarantism existed in the mid-twentieth century. His focus on tarantism as a cultural phenomenon questioned psychologically determined interpretations, unveiling the personal crises of the tarantate as symptomatic of larger conflicts on a social level. De Martino drew on the work of the politician and philosopher Antonio Gramsci to depict the conflict between the hegemonic order, the 'capitalist form of domination through ideas rather than through the use of force' (Saunders 1984: 455), and the subaltern, 'subordinate, proletarian and rural proletarian' (ibid.) classes, to which the majority of the tarantate belonged. In this sense, *La terra del rimorso* was ideologically motivated by De Martino's belief in 'the "historicization" of the subaltern world as a prophylactic against … exploitation' (ibid.: 456). This study was, moreover, embedded within a larger intellectual context, in which De Martino became a founding figure of Italian ethnology (although he saw himself primarily as a historian of religion), influenced by philosophical and political currents of post-war Italy, and specifically the ideas of Benedetto Croce and Antonio Gramsci, (Gallini 1982; Lorenzetti 1982; Saunders 1984). De Martino's contribution to studies on southern Italy was fundamental in revealing that alleviating the enormous differences between southern and northern Italy required not only economic engagement, but also initiatives promoting a rebirth of the South on a cultural level.

La terra del rimorso was a prime example. It proposed a new approach to southern Italy's situation. The magico-religious perspective of its protagonists was examined not as an evolutionary relic of primitive thinking, but as a culturally specific response to harsh living conditions. De Martino proposed a psychoanalytically tinged interpretation viewed within a historical and socio-economic framework. Tarantism was defined as a 'religion of remorse', allowing for the payment of debts contracted on an existential level. The tarantula was employed as a symbol for eliciting traumatic experiences of the past, many of these linked to the recurring themes of forbidden love, unfulfilled desires and repressed emotions. The ritual of tarantism became a means for reliving and healing individual crises threatening to explode without control. It served as a channel of expression and resolution according to a historically proven and socially acknowledged model.

Tarantism, according to De Martino, was irreducible to any form of spider poisoning. The tarantula was a mythical spider, an ideological complex autonomous in its symbolism as it explained the symptoms of the tarantate even in the absence of an actual bite. Few of De Martino's interviewees had, in fact, suffered from a real spider bite. All, however, appeared to suffer from a 'crisis of presence' at the time of their initial affliction: a sense of the self as unreal and unrelated to present circumstances, implying a loss of referents in the surrounding world, often in the face of socio-economic and natural calamities (De Martino 1956, 1960, 1975; Pandolfi 1990). Disaster struck and fuses blew, snapping the relational threads that linked a healthy individual to her or his body, community and environment.

It was here that the tarantula intervened. Through the injection of its poison, De Martino explains, the mystic spider transferred its attributes to its victim. Many became melancholic, others aggressive or highly erotic in their behaviour. On average, three or four days of dancing, especially to the rhythmic sounds of the pizzica tarantata, provided the only way out. The rhythmic order of sounds, argues De Martino, not only released tensions into movements, but also provided 'a very elementary cultural order to be preferentially relied upon when a great existential catastrophe loomed' (2005: 94).

Overall, research on tarantism following *La terra del rimorso* (De Martino 1961a) has built on this rich contribution without challenging it extensively. Nevertheless, various critiques have been voiced. Some demanded further contextualization of the socio-economic and political situation of southern Italy in the 1950s (Cassin 1962: 133; Lorenzetti 1982: 28–31) and of the relationship between those participating in the ideology of tarantism and those discounting it as a superstition (Lorenzetti 1982: 28–31). Historians challenged De Martino's search for tarantism's origins in Greek Dionysian cults (Lapassade 1994; Di Mitri 1996; Horden 2000) and added to or questioned his historical sources (Turchini 1987; Salvatore 2000; Vallone 2004; Di Mitri 2006). Others pointed out that the mythico-ritualistic complex of tarantism was not considered in relation to the larger context of traditional curative practices (Coppa 1996: 31) and, by dismissing the psychopathological approach as inherently reductive, De Martino failed to recognize that psychiatry was increasingly broadening its parameters to include sociocultural variables (Anon. 1967: 347). A focus on the symbolic level and its possible roots in ancient Greek traditions has, moreover, obscured the importance of the performative element, based on identification with the tarantula spider (Rouget 1986: 161), and of broader performance contexts, including related healing rituals or festive occasions (Lüdtke 2000b). Some of these gaps were addressed in subsequent research.

Recent Studies: Continuing the Quest for Answers

De Martino and his team were generally welcomed, it seems, into the houses of the tarantate. Many participated in interviews hoping that the medically qualified researchers would find alternative forms of relief for their misery. The publication of *La terra del rimorso* brought crowds of curious visitors to the Salento. In June every year, the town of Galatina was swamped with film crews and photographers. For many journalists and researchers, the Salento became an exotic location still harbouring pagan relics, which needed to be documented at all costs prior to extinction. Many condemned the tarantate's performances as tourist enterprises staged purely for collecting money. At the same time, many benefited from the image Galatina gained as a pilgrimage site. Every year, masses of visitors spent their lire at local hotels, shops and market stalls (Panico 1983: 55–91). They also increasingly met with the tarantate's resistance to be interviewed or filmed (Montinaro 1976: 72).

In the wake of *La terra del rimorso*, research on tarantism can, for the sake of convenience, be subdivided into three general themes, socio-economic, medical and anthropological, depending on the key focus taken. Studies on the socio-economic context of tarantism tended both to elaborate on aspects neglected by De Martino and to document and analyse tarantism's transformations in subsequent years. Medically inclined research refined the psychologically reductive analyses criticized by De Martino. Tarantism was inserted into a history of medicine and compared to other therapeutic systems that challenged the incompatibility of biologically and socially determined interpretations, although some psychologically reductive studies persisted. Most anthropological studies were characterized by a comparative approach. In particular, studies in psychological anthropology have been central in weaving tarantism into a broader fabric of healing rites interpreted in terms of spirit possession and altered states of consciousness. This section presents a chronological synthesis and selection of research based on both textual and cinematographic sources, showing that these three fields are neither mutually exclusive nor exhaustive. Moreover, the studies considered are limited to the Salento and to tarantism as understood in its ancient, ritual sense.[9] No reference is made at this point to studies on the contemporary revitalization of the tarantula's music and dance.[10]

Studies considered here as socio-economic were often of high ethnographic import, providing valuable descriptions of the general living conditions of the tarantate. Perhaps the most famous and insightful of these was anthropologist Annabella Rossi's book *Lettere da una tarantata*, Letters from a tarantata (1970), based on her correspondence with a tarantata in the Salento over a six-year period from 1959 to 1965. These letters recurrently touched on the harshness of existing living conditions based on agricultural labour, the anxieties linked to being a woman in tight-knit family circles, and the hopes and prayers invested in religious figures appealed to for well-being. The tarantata who dictated these letters suffered from epileptic fits from an early age and identified the cause for these in two different maladies – one attributed to St Paul and the other to St Donatus – which she distinguished according to whether she felt the urge to dance or not: only St Paul required her to do so. The publication of these letters remains a unique testimony of a tarantata's life conveyed in her own voice, without, however, escaping the dilemmas of representation: inevitably these letters were edited and existed in relation to Rossi's own letters.[11]

Writing a few years later, Brizio Montinaro (1976) described tarantism as a rusty tool of the past, still deeply rooted among parts of the Salentine community. He suggested that the option of tarantism may have stood in the way of potentially urgent medical intervention, after witnessing how a young man, subsequently diagnosed with a brain tumour, was brought to St Paul's chapel in Galatina. This view of tarantism as a two-sided sword was further exposed in a valuable article by Miriam Castiglione and Luciana Stocchi (1977). Their Marxist-inspired study took a close look at the lives of the tarantate in relation to those who did not share their belief system. It focused particularly on the ecclesiastical and socio-political context, as well as the condition of women, in the 1970s Salento. The domestic exploitation of female labour, seen within a framework of capitalist development, rural depopulation and emigration, revealed how many women were left to rely on limited family and neighbourhood contacts, as well as the mass media, to overcome situations of extreme social isolation. At the same time, the religious ideology inherent in the insertion of Pauline theology into tarantism rituals perpetuated the exploitation of women as reproducers of the existing labour force and as substitutes for insufficient social services. The Christian influence on tarantism was unveiled as fostering the causes of the tarantate's misery, despite the temporary relief conceded by pilgrimages to Galatina.

In the early 1980s, the documentary film *Morso d'amore* (Miscuglio et al. 1981) threw into relief changes in both the socio-economic context and the performance techniques of tarantism. The film-makers documented a case of self-instigated therapy: images of a tarantata rocking from side to side on her bed, singing to herself, invoking the presence of St Paul and the tarantula. No musicians were involved and only one other participant sat by the side of her bed to ensure that she did not come to any harm. This woman was bitten on her first day back at work in the fields of the Salento after years of factory labour (and better working conditions) in Switzerland. She told the camera that her periods had ceased from this day onwards and returned only when she finally received St Paul's grace, the very year she became the protagonist of *Morso d'amore*. We may dismiss this link as a mere coincidence or question what impact the camera team may have had on her life. Was its presence enough to render her misery public, visible to the eyes of others, and hence imaginable, acceptable and possible to process?

A comparison to Ada's performance for the Canale 5 cameras, twenty years later, inevitably comes to mind. Both told their story in verbal and corporal form, sustained by the gaze of others, human eyes and camera lenses, acknowledging and recording it in tangible form. As their fate was aired and made public, legitimate, so to speak, potential sentiments of shame, embarrassment or guilt are likely to have lost their charge, becoming redundant, suggesting a step towards recovery. Historically, too, tarantism rituals were characterized by their public nature. This case was, moreover, not the only one to involve a returning emigrant. Just one year later, Gianfranco Mingozzi, in his film *Sulla terra del rimorso* (1982), documented a similar case of a tarantato who was bitten when settling once again in the Salento after years of working abroad. It is also significant that many of those who passionately brought about the revitalization of the pizzica in the 1990s had spent some time working or studying in northern Italy, France, Switzerland, Germany or elsewhere before returning home to the Salento.

Medical perspectives on tarantism, meanwhile, variously engaged the views of ethnopsychiatry, the history of medicine, psychoanalysis, medical anthropology, toxicology and music therapy. Ethnopsychiatric work on tarantism brought into relief problems of defining psychopathologies, as the cause of the tarantate's afflictions was sought in both biological and social terms. Psychiatrist Giovanni Jervis (1961, 1962) argued that biologically defined symptoms of psychosis and schizophrenia could be detected in some tarantate, but, nevertheless, tarantism had to be seen as an ideological institution: as a culturally specific instrument of explanation, used to define and alleviate symptoms irreducible to any one interpretative schema. George Mora (1963) addressed these issues by considering tarantism in relation to the diagnosis of psychopathologies in ancient Greek culture and contemporary psychotherapy. Piero Coppa (1996: 29–33), referring to De Martino (1961a), as well as to Risso and Böker's study (1964) on psychopathologies among South Italian migrant workers in Switzerland, emphasized the danger of stigmatizing individuals by using out of context terminology.

Research on the link between actual spider bites and tarantism has been scarce. Eric Carlson and Meredith Simpson's study (1971) of a nineteenth-century case in America provided one exception: it told of a young woman from Rhode Island bitten by a tarantula for whom the only effective treatment proved to be music and dancing. In this case, the ritual of tarantism may well have been unknown to the young female victim and it is unclear what other factors may have come into play. Historian Peregrine Horden (2000: 251) suggested that a translation of Giorgio Baglivi's (1696) book, printed in the *New York Magazine* of 1797, and 'the physician's unwitting power of suggestion' may have had a prominent role in this choice of treatment. More recently, in 1996, a case of spider poisoning was registered in the Salento and carefully documented by the doctors involved (Colonna et al. 1997, 2000). It revealed a close analogy between the symptoms of actual spider poisoning and those of the tarantate. Although insufficient case studies of actual spider bites exist in the Salento to be able to draw well-founded parallels, it was inevitably noted that the symptoms of this young patient subsided after three to four days, the average period of dancing required for the ritual of tarantism (Chiriatti 1997b).[12]

Psychoanalytical studies of tarantism focused on the sexual symbolism inherent in these rituals. Psychiatrist Dario Caggia (1984) made a unique reference to a tarantata subjected to psychoanalysis. Unfortunately, few, if any, insights were given about this treatment; instead, symbolic references to Greek myths were drawn upon to provide an interpretative context. A provocative, although little developed, stance on the relation between tarantism and sexuality was taken by Luigi Chiriatti and Georges Lapassade (1985) in the context of Salentine performance traditions more generally, considering music-making and dancing as a means of socially evoking, expressing and controlling individual erotic impulses.

Historian of medicine Angelo Turchini (1987) provided an extensive review of medical literature on tarantism, creating a valuable complement to *La terra del rimorso*. His focus was on the use of therapeutic elements, particularly music, songs, conjurations and the role of healing figures, such as the *sanpaolari*, putative descendants of St Paul said to have healing qualities, and the *capo-attarantati*, responsible for conducting tarantism rituals. On an interpretative level, Turchini equated tarantism with linguistic alchemy, a system of explanation facilitated by the use of non-verbal media. Meanwhile, Jean Russell's (1979) medical history of tarantism continued to define this phenomenon as a form of hysteria particular to the Mediterranean context.

With regard to the field of the performance arts therapies and particularly music therapy, tarantism has been prized as an early European example of this discipline (Alvin 1966; Horden 2000) and simultaneously dismissed as an obstacle to the professional recognition of the arts therapies. Various studies considering the relationship between music and medicine in historical and cross-cultural contexts have touched on the tradition of tarantism (Schullian and Schoen 1948; Kümmel 1977; Tomlinson 1994; Gouk 2000; Horden 2000). Interestingly, Kümmel (1977: 21), in his detailed and lengthy summary of examples of music and medicine in (primarily European) contexts of 800–1800, deliberately refused to take tarantism and related dancing mania into account, considering them to be inappropriate to the context of humoral medicine. His explanation was that, whereas medical practitioners applied music to regulate and balance patients' moods, the so-called dance epidemics accentuated existing moods, thereby not helping to attain an emotional equilibrium.[13]

Medical anthropology, meanwhile, has emphasized the importance of indigenous illness contexts, categories and meanings. Robert Bartholomew contested the widespread classification of tarantism as a form of mass psychogenic illness, which, he argued, 'may involve normal, rational people who possess unfamiliar conduct codes, worldviews and political agendas that differ significantly from those of Western-trained investigators' (1994: 281). This article showed how universal categories inevitably succumb to cultural prejudices, thereby uncovering reductive stances. Vittorio Lanternari (1995, 2000) considered tarantism with reference to religious healing rituals, arguing that these were not so much directed at combating clinically definable states of psychophysical illness, but rather worked towards overcoming experiences of suffering linked to psychosomatic syndromes: sensations of emptiness and a lack of points of reference and meaning to life. Drawing comparisons between tarantism and two charismatic healing cults, his focus was on the performative use of the body. Physical enactments were considered a means of accessing a symbolic world and activating the body's auto-therapeutic potential. Lanternari's work suggested that symptoms of tarantism persisted despite the decline of this tradition, and underlined the risk of categorizing and treating certain human conditions as forms of illness when these may be inherently auto-therapeutic.

A comparative approach has also characterized anthropological studies, developing De Martino's (2005: 177–86) references to ethnographic, folkloric and historical parallels of tarantism. Bringing into play relations of power and gender, Ioan Lewis (1971) defined tarantism as a form of rebellion and possession determined by social marginality. Tarantism was presented as an aggressive strategy for the politically impotent, predominantly women and occasionally men, constrained to live in socially oppressive circumstances. Entry into this protest cult, an integral part of the therapeutic process, was achieved by succumbing to the mythical tarantula's illness. Although personal situations may not be radically remedied, Lewis argued, relief was found in a 'religious idiom, which men can condone as a divinely sanctioned therapy' (1971: 92). Along similar lines, in his cross-cultural study on the role of music in triggering states of trance, Gilbert Rouget (1986) argued that tarantism was a means for the public expression of hysteria, facilitating recovery through bodily imitation with the source of affliction. Rouget, moreover, emphasized that tarantism was not a form of exorcism, 'not a conflictual relation with the deity that is involved, but the partaking of an alliance' (1986: 164): the spider and that which it symbolized were appeased rather than expelled. For this reason, the diverse performative ways of identifying and coming to terms with the spider were crucial. Georges Lapassade's (1994, 1996a, b, 2001) research, meanwhile, has aimed at retrieving the meaning of trance rituals as a human resource for use in modern contexts. Inserting tarantism into this line of research, he emphasized its affinity with Corybante dances as opposed to Dionysian rituals, describing the experience of performers in trance rituals as based on the explosion of an ordinary state of consciousness resulting from the rhythmic synchrony established between musicians and performers.

A reading of these studies provokes critiques associated with the choice of terms used to refer to subjective experiences and notions of consciousness. It raises questions about the wide range of definitions applied to so-called altered states, about what is seen to induce these and how they are experienced and explained in culturally specific terms. Moreover, these issues bring into play difficulties of establishing criteria of ethnographic and/or biomedical authenticity and genuineness, which may not only overlap but also include various levels and ways of talking about these terms (Hamayon 1995; Becker 2004). In the Salento, these problems are magnified, as many – both performers and researchers – uncritically use the Italian terms *trance* and *stati alterati* or *modificati di coscienza* to describe experiences of music-making or dancing, thereby enhancing risks of covering up culturally and individually specific forms of expression with standardized labels.

Such reflections have led Damian Walter (2000: 112–13) to propose an alternative, without, however, escaping the hazards of generalization:

> In preference to terms such as trance, ecstasy and altered or alternate states
> of consciousness ... the notion of an *altered state of awareness* ... gives

support to the idea that in a culturally-recognized 'trance' state – however defined – the subject learns to identify and give precedence to different visual, aural, somatic, and mental criteria, without necessarily implying that he or she becomes dissociated from his or her immediate surroundings and without prioritizing etic categories concerned with the truth or falsity of what is believed to be taking place.

With regard to the anthropology of performance, little research on tarantism is available. Luigi Santoro (1982, 1987) has approached tarantism through his own experience of theatre. Likewise, Michela Almiento (1990) set out to discuss Joseph Moreno's ideas on psychodrama in relation to the tarantate's rituals, but did not pursue this perspective beyond the confines of her master's thesis. Some significant contributions to historical and contemporary interpretations of tarantism were provided in two volumes of conference papers published as a result of the international conference *Quarant'anni dopo De Martino* (Forty years after De Martino) in October 1998 (Di Mitri 2000). Experiences and accounts of the world of tarantism in the last few decades have, moreover, been published in various recent books by Giorgio Di Lecce (1994), Luigi Chiriatti (1995) and Maurizio Nocera (2005) and are also portrayed in Edoardo Winspeare's documentary *San Paolo e la tarantola* (1989).[14] These studies document the persistence of tarantism on the margins of contemporary life and public health care in the 1980s and 1990s despite constant declarations of its extinction. This paradox appears central to the multiple and changing manifestations of contemporary tarantism.

Notes

1. Ernesto De Martino (2005: 214–15) cites this account from Malaterra (1724). According to Jean Russell (1979: 405), Ardoini also refers to earlier writers, such as Avicenna, Rhazes, Gilbert the Englishman, Albucasis and others, who wrote about the cure of the tarantula's bite.

2. For a discussion of similarities and differences between tarantism and St Vitus's and St John's dances, see also Katner (1956: 77–82) and De Martino (2005: 217–22).

3. For a discussion of the symbolic links between ancient Greek cults and tarantism, see De Martino (2005: 187–211) and Salvatore (1989: 217–45). Lapassade (1994: 10) focuses on tarantism's similarities to the Corybante rites and Di Mitri (1996: 11–28) has emphasized the Orphic connection to tarantism.

4. See also Horden (2003) on issues of historical continuity and discontinuity with respect to music therapy in the Mediterranean more generally.

5. See Ovid's *Metamorphoses* (1957), Book VI. Pierpaolo De Giorgi (1999: 176) draws an analogy to the legend of Sanarica by positing a link between the evil woman (Arachne) and the Virgin (Athena).

6. For references to the history of tarantism, see Sigerist (1948: 96–116); Katner (1956: 5–25); Mora (1963: 417–39); Turchini (1987); Chiriatti (1995: 31–46); Baldwin (1997: 163–91); Convegno (1999); Gentilcore (2000); De Martino (2005: 187–244); Di Mitri (2006).

7. For reprints of these historical texts, see Lüdtke (2000b: 318–27).

8. The team members included Giovanni Jervis (psychiatrist); Letizia Jervis-Comba (psychologist); Diego Carpitella (ethnomusicologist); Amalia Signorelli D'Ayala (social anthropologist); and Vittoria De Palma (social assistant).

9. For research on tarantism in Spain and Campania, see León Sanz (2000, 2008) and Rossi (1991) respectively; for studies on the related phenomenon of the *argia* in Sardinia, see Gallini (1967, 1988).

10. See Nacci (2001, 2004); De Giorgi (2002, 2005); Lamanna (2002); Santoro and Torsello (2002); Collu (2005); Del Giudice and van Deusen (2005); Durante (2005); Thayer (2005); Imbriani and Fumarola (2007).

11. Paolo Apolito (1994) edited a further edition, showing what new light recent anthropological developments throw on this correspondence. Anna's case has also been analysed from a psychoanalytical perspective by Francesco Lazzari (1972: 91–134).

12. See Chapter 3, 'Spider Poisoning: a Contested Case'.

13. For a review, see Peregrine Horden (2000: 21–40).

14. Winspeare subsequently went on to produce two further fictional films linked to the tarantula's music and dance: *Pizzicata* (1994), a wartime love story involving a case of tarantism, and *Sangue Vivo* (2000), the story of two brothers involved in smuggling and drugs, inspired by the true story of Salentine tambourine player Pino Zimba.

Part II
The Spider's Cult Today

In the contemporary Salento, the living webs of old and new tarantati intersect, the first frail, dismissed and practically abandoned, the second neon-bright and vibrant. Part II is an ethnographic journey following the tarantula's tracks across both types of web. Chapter 3, 'Curing Myths and Fictive Cures', looks at old-time silver-threaded webs of the world of tarantism. It juxtaposes the views of believers and sceptics, bringing spiders alive and killing them off as they speak. Novel expressions of the tarantula's dance reveal new web designs, as Chapter 4, 'Ads and Antidotes', confirms. From backstage circles of musicians and dancers to satellite-broadcast mega-concerts, the tarantula today weaves its web across the globe and broader spatial orbits. As a multi-purpose toolkit, music and dance have become a potent logo of Salentine identity, serving both to accentuate conflict and to bring about a sense of community. They present a choice, a very visible and audible one, between taking opposition or joining forces and the manifold options in between. Whereas historically music was the only antidote for the tarantate, the same notes function today as tourist ads and fun fair invites. Chapter 5, 'Sensing Identities and Well-being', proceeds to consider personal accounts, showing how the spotlights on today's buzz around the tarantula's music and dance can serve to blind us to the sociocultural implications of contemporary afflictions and to re-appropriated discourses on healing and well-being.

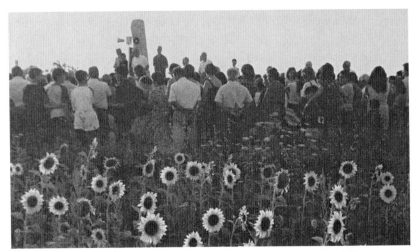

Fig. 3.1 Mass at the grotto of St Paul in Giurdignano, June 1998 (photo: Fernando Bevilacqua).

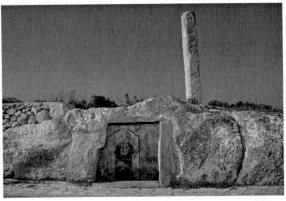

Figs 3.2 and 3.3 The Giurdignano grotto with the fresco of St Paul next to the tarantula's web, September 2007 (photos: Erhard Söhner).

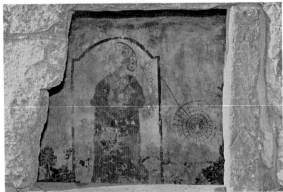

Chapter 3
Curing Myths and Fictive Cures: Views of Believers and Sceptics

> There is a Salento that believes
> in the tambourine, in music,
> and there is a Salento that does not believe.
> Today, tarantism is this.
>
> Galatina, 23 June 1999[1]

In its ancient, curative sense, tarantism has become extinct. Public rituals of music and dance, once widespread throughout the Salentine peninsula, Apulia and beyond, no longer exist. This fact is well-known and open to little doubt. And yet the belief system within which this ritual dance was wrapped has not dissolved into time immemorial. A minority of believers and a majority of sceptics reside side by side in the Salento today. This was sharply brought home to me one afternoon in August 1999 when I talked to two elderly gentlemen in the south-west of the Salento. One, a victim of the tarantula, had been at the mercy of the spider's whims for three consecutive years in the 1960s. The other, a fervent scholar of tarantism, was convinced that this ritual tradition was nothing but pretence, theatre and fiction. These two perspectives, indicative of the tensions between believers and sceptics more generally, continue to clash as they have done for centuries.

Tarantism as Cure: Debates in Favour of the Tarantula

It is 11 August 1999 and the five o'clock afternoon heat is stifling in the kitchen of Francesco Greco's apartment. We sit around a large table above which a ceiling fan is stirring the humid air. My brain is numb from the heat and sweat runs down my legs, with a cotton skirt creating sauna conditions. It takes every bit of concentration to hold onto the thread of questions prepared in my mind for this interview, at risk of being swept away by the centrifugal force of the rotating blades above our heads. I have come with two personal contacts, Vittorio Marras and Bengasi Fai, thanks to whom this meeting was arranged. We sit down at the long kitchen table with Francesco. His wife Cinzia and a young woman and child settle down on a sofa nearby. They form a backdrop to the scene, with Francesco's wife taking an active, almost sentinel-like part in the conversation. I ask how everything started.[2]

Francesco:	I don't remember the year. It was some twenty years ago.[3]
Karen:	And was it a spider?
Francesco:	I can't tell you that it was a spider. It's also possible that it was a snake or a scorpion.
Karen:	Did you feel the bite?
Francesco:	Yes, I felt it. I was working where the grain was being ground and I felt something sting me, but didn't really take notice of it. I continued to work. At the moment of the bite, you don't feel anything. Then, after a day or two, I began to feel unwell and vomited. The vomit was yellow, like the poison that this animal was carrying.
Karen:	And what did you feel?
Francesco:	My body felt completely abandoned,[4] tired and very heavy. You couldn't even take a cup into your hands. I now pick up a quintal,[5] but then not even a cup. It wasn't clear what it was or what this affliction depended on.[6] The doctors didn't find anything. They didn't find a poison internally. We went to see major specialists, but they never found anything. They told me to have an injection and gave me one, but there was nothing to do, because it was that problem, that illness which the saint gave me. There are no medicines that can cure you. And they don't find anything wrong, because we are healthy. As persons we are completely healthy.
Karen:	But you weren't well.

Francesco: I wasn't well at all. The doctors call us mad. When you speak about certain things, about these illnesses, the doctors say: 'Nothing of this is true!' The doctors don't believe. Our own family doctor says that we're staging a show for people. That's why those other people came to play. After a day, two days, or even a week – there are people who danced for a week and even two weeks – you received the saint's grace. Now some of the doctors believe, not all of them, but some. It's because now they have begun to study these things, the new doctors.

Karen: And how did you know what the affliction was?

Francesco: Those who played the music had come across many others with this illness. The doctors didn't believe in this illness, but my family, my mother, my father, the other people said: 'It must be the tarantula! It must be the tarantula!' Word got round that I wasn't well. In this state, we don't want to go outside and are always in bed, feeling abandoned like that. And the people asked: 'How come?' If someone in the village isn't well, word gets round immediately. And people said: 'It must be the tarantula.' I had an aunt, my mother's sister, who played the tambourine. She came round one day, on her own, without telling me or anyone else. She came secretly and brought the tambourine and started to play, just the tambourine, on her own. When I heard the tambourine, I started … And that's when my aunt said: 'It's the tarantula!' She had seen hundreds, hundreds of these cases and so when she saw me in this condition, she knew.

    The next day my aunt called the musicians. There were three. I didn't know anything about this, as I was in bed, feeling completely abandoned. They came to my mother's and prepared the house. They put covers on the floor, because when we fall, we fall and can end up hitting a chair or the wall. The musicians came around 11, 11.30 a.m. and started to play for ten minutes, for fifteen minutes. The music made me react on the bed, jump up, dance. I got out of bed on my own and went to the room next door and danced.

    There were also some colours that bothered me, because there are certain colours that the animal doesn't like. The animal chooses the colour. At Galatina, we were capable of stripping someone of their jacket or vest because we didn't like the colour. One woman remained naked in the middle of the street. If the animal was yellow, then it was yellow that it couldn't bear seeing. Or red. And we were the same. We would always look out for this colour.

Karen: What instruments were there?

Francesco: There was a tambourine, a diatonic accordion and a violin.[7] Not an accordion, but a diatonic accordion, because the accordion doesn't give you the same sound. It was important that it was this diatonic accordion, because, if someone took up the accordion, the music wasn't the same. With the tambourine it is the same. If someone just plays, you don't feel anything. I can tell if it's played by someone who is an expert, who plays the beat of that music, of that illness. You can tell if someone is competent in those things.

Karen: And did they know what to play, or did you ask for specific music?

Francesco: No, no, no, they played the sound of the tarantula, of that animal. Even today they play that sound of the tarantula. There are tapes. Even though I like that music, and I buy it for myself at times, after a little while, I turn it off. It's the only music that I really like, because of the grace that I received. But I immediately sweat, because I still feel a little bit this event of some thirty years ago. They used to play one hour, two hours, depending on what the saint said. There has to be a person that commands us, and it may be that it is this saint. You see an image. While we dance, we see a person in front of us. But we don't know who this person is. We see a shadow. It's he who commands you. He tells you what you have to do and what you don't have to do. In my sister's case, it was a snake. But with her it took just one year.

Karen: And, for you, how long did it take?

Francesco: Three, four years, no? For one or two days you were really in a bad state and then there was this vision, this person that said: 'You don't have to dance any more. Enough!'

Karen: Did others perceive this vision?

Francesco: No, no one.

Cinzia: Some people were told by the saint to go around the village to collect offerings.

Francesco: One year my sister said that she needed one hundred, two hundred thousand lire[8] and we were ready to give them to her to take to the saint, but my sister said: 'No'. She had to collect these as offerings. She had to go down the streets to collect this money. My mother said that we had this money to give, but the saint didn't accept. Previously, you heard a lot about these things, and people believed in these things and more than one gave a thousand lire, five hundred lire, and the sum of money collected was enough to go to Galatina and to offer to the saint. The priest then took the money, or someone else took it. Once my sister had collected this money and gone to Galatina, she was all well again, completely fine.

Then the last year that I did this, after two, three days always in these conditions, this vision said that the following day was the day of St Peter and Paul. We generally went the day before. I went to do my duty, but he sent me away. The saint, this shadow, said to me: 'You shouldn't have come today. You have to come back. You have to come tomorrow.' I had to turn back, to go back home, in a bad state, to wake up at four in the morning and to return on foot. My brother, my father, my mother wanted to take me by car. But he said: 'No, I won't accept.' I had to go on foot and left on my own.

Cinzia: I'll never forget the last year that he was really ill, in 1967. Of course we were worried at home. I followed him secretly by car, to see in case he wasn't well, but I just wasn't able to see him anywhere. Who knows which road he took.

Francesco: They didn't see me. But I was on the road. It's not that I took another road. I took the normal road to Galatina, the principal road. And they say that they didn't see me. I took one hour to get to Galatina and close to the church my family saw me. It's possible that they passed by me and didn't see me. When I arrived, I went to the small church, because you have to go first to the small church and then to the large church. I had to move on my knees from the chapel to the large church. It's about a hundred metres distant. The altar was all laid out with people all around and I don't know how I found myself there, but I found myself on the statue of St Paul.

Karen: On the statue?

Francesco: I found myself on the statue of St Paul in the church.

Karen: On top?

Francesco: On top. I don't know how I got there, how I climbed up onto the statue. Then the police arrived and other people. They thought I was mad, because the saint carries a golden angel and they thought that I'd gone up there to steal the gold. I arrived on top of the saint and then came down by myself. The priests condemned me, but I didn't hear anything, I didn't see anything. I didn't even see the police or the people inside the church. The people in Galatina don't believe in these things. They don't believe, because at Galatina St Peter and Paul have protected their territory, saying that here these things should not exist.

In the whole province this happens, but not in Galatina. In most parts, there were one or two per village. I met many of these people. Most of them are dead now. Among the young, few have remained. I have remained alone with these things. But in the church you still find these people, old ones, aged eighty or so, and they still do these tricks.[9] These people still dance. In the church, you need to close the door, because, you know, a man wears trousers, but a woman doesn't and there are people who don't believe in these things and they come to look, to laugh, to joke. Also, at the back of this church, there was a cistern with water inside and it was full of snakes. There was a bucket with which you brought up the water. Those of us who suffered from this affliction drank, but no other person did. When the water came up in the bucket, those serpents, and scorpions – I don't know which animals they were, because you didn't see them – disappeared inside the bucket and just water came out. Not everyone could drink this water, but we drank it without worries.

Karen: And what about the music?

Francesco: There were people who played music inside the church. The musicians who played were brought by the family from one's own village.

Karen: And what effect did the music have?

Francesco: You felt stronger. You felt things the force of which even we didn't know how to explain. You saw serpents. You saw people thread themselves through chairs,[10] without even noticing. I'd never manage now, but then I did. And I was always big as I am now. But, it wasn't me. It was all based on this animal that did all of these things.

Cinzia: There was no control on their part. They can't perceive why they did it or how they managed to do it. The point is that they don't even remember.

Karen: And this shadow, did it appear when the affliction began?[11]

Francesco: First you had the affliction and you danced to this music. Then, when you were feeling tired, you asked for grace from this saint because you just couldn't take it any more, because you felt just too tired. You asked for the saint's grace and he told you what to do, depending on the penance that you had to fulfil, depending on the effect of this poison, of this animal.

Karen: And why was it St Paul?

Francesco: St Paul is our protector. It was he who directed me. He is the person in the vision that we have. It's just that we don't know who it is. We imagine that it is this saint. And we speak with him. You don't hear anything. I spoke with myself, and the saint. There was no one else who could hear. I could even speak in a loud voice, but the people around couldn't hear anything.

Bengasi:	Before, had you ever thought about this saint?
Francesco:	No, to be honest, I never went to visit St Peter and Paul. When I was young, I went to St Pantaleon, because my father took me to the festival. He was a devotee of St Pantaleon. I never thought about these saints. Afterwards, yes. Before, in fact, at times I'd use the saints' names in blasphemy. Nowadays, if I hear someone who speaks badly of St Paul, I immediately get furious. I feel uneasy, because they are referring to this saint. For me this saint is a confidential thing, and, if others don't show proper respect for him, I get very angry. I have been fortunate with this saint. For those of us who have this illness, who have been bitten by this illness, we have all been saved. I believe in this saint, because he is a saint that has made me well. Thank God, he granted me health.
Cinzia:	Were you there at St Peter and Paul's?
Karen:	Yes.
Cinzia:	(*turning towards me*): So you were there in the chapel. We were coming out and you arrived and sat down. In fact, I said: 'That's someone who's interested, let's go.' I said: 'Please, hurry up, let's get out of here,' that's what I said, 'There's someone from the RAI,[12] when here there are people who aren't well.' ... You sat down on the small bench near to the wall. And I said: 'Let's go. Let's go.' (*Her emotional tone encourages me to come to an end, despite Francesco's invitation to ask as many questions as we liked.*)
Karen:	One last question, when you received grace, how did you feel?
Francesco:	Well. Normal. I left the church, went to the bar and had a coffee, as if nothing had happened. For three years, I was unwell. Throughout the year, I was fine until this period arrived. But since I have received this final grace, following my visit on foot to Galatina, I have found myself well. But I still go to the church every year to do my duty, and as soon as I arrive near the small church, I feel emotional because I think everything might come back once again.

Francesco continues to speak long after I have switched off my tape recorder. My companions and I stand in his kitchen, in his doorway, and then outside his house, next to the car, gripped by his accounts, unable to leave. The memories triggered by our visit pour forth. His speech is passionate. It holds us, preventing us from turning on the car's ignition, inhibiting us from bidding him farewell. It is as if this tale is seeking to keep our attention so as to be spun on, so as not to be suspended or abandoned in the air. It is a long while before we eventually depart, and I wonder what repercussions our visit has had on Francesco's life and that of his family. It seemed as if our coming had stirred deep waters, yet again recalling emotions of crises brought on by the tarantula. I can't help but wonder what events had led to Francesco's affliction, what human relations created the backdrop to his crises, and how others involved might have presented his case. I never did find out.

In spite of this obvious partiality, Francesco's account is that of a believer: although he was no longer subject to the tarantula's sting, the return of its symptoms was always, potentially, imminent. This conviction does not belong to Francesco alone, although the tarantate persisting today are a tiny minority. Others confirm their existence, although accounts of their well-being vary. In 1998, Luigi Chiriatti, well-known for his research on popular music and Salentine traditions, confirmed the following during a seminar at the University of Lecce: 'There are still some fifteen tarantate that I know in the Salento today who are suffering from the symptoms of tarantism. Some continue to perform rituals in the privacy of their homes. None, however, directly and openly admit that they are tarantate.'[13] On the same day, Salentine writer Maurizio Nocera explained: 'There are still some tarantate who are "performing" in their homes today. Until the day before yesterday, Christina performed the rituals you see in the film *Morso d'amore*.[14] Now she is in hospital because she is not well … You will find that most of these individuals do not talk.' By 2006, Nocera estimated that there were no more than five or six tarantate still alive.[15] Meanwhile, social anthropologist Stephen Bennetts (2006) writes: 'According to one Salentine authority, the last episode of tarantism took place in 1993, and the last living practitioner died in 2000.' Clearly, there is much room for speculation.

Personally, I have met no more than five (ex)tarantate during my time in the Salento and I am unable to confirm the persistence of any rituals involving music and dance. However, like Francesco and Evelina, a number of tarantate continue their pilgrimages to Galatina in commemoration of St Paul in June every year. It is here that public performances of tarantism were still observed in the early 1990s (Almiento 1990; Di Lecce 1994). These accounts are variously disputed and sometimes dismissed as nothing but show, as researchers' attempts at seeking credit and recognition. Personally, I have no proof for the date of the most recent performance at Galatina. However, in my interviews various unconnected accounts of these rituals in the early 1990s confirm one another.[16]

However this may be, this site too appears to be increasingly abandoned, perhaps replaced, and certainly reinvented, as Matteo's dance in June 2001 suggests. Luigi Santoro (1982: 75), professor of theatre history at the University of Lecce, meanwhile, hints at the fact that ritual pilgrimages have been displaced to other sites in the Salentine countryside:

> Michelina … told me that the following year she would no longer come to Galatina; like the other tarantate, she too would go to … If you want to come – she had added – come alone. Each year we count ourselves to see who has remained and who has died … But don't bring anybody else, otherwise the black tarantula will take revenge and eat us all.

On 29 June 2007, a young researcher from Ostuni suggests the same as we chat in the chapel of St Paul. To my knowledge, these hints have not been followed up or mentioned in writing elsewhere, although another landmark, St Paul's grotto, just outside the town of Giurdignano, sees St Paul and the tarantula spider venerated side by side.

St Paul's Grotto: a Contested Site

For most of the year, this grotto is bare except for moss and fern growing inside its moist ecosphere [see Figs 3.2 and 3.3]. The months of May and June bring change, as the crypt interior fills up with red-glowing candles, bouquets of wheat, potted plants and fresh wild flowers. By the time St Paul's feast day arrives, much of the cavern floor is covered with offerings. On 29 June 1998, I attended a service here [see Fig. 3.1].

By seven o'clock in the evening, a crowd of about seventy people has flocked around St Paul's grotto. It is surrounded by fields of sunflowers and lies some hundred metres beyond the periphery of the town of Giurdignano on the convex curve of a tarred country road. Painted on the faded walls inside the cavern are two human figures and a spider web: it is here that St Paul dwells side by side with the tarantula. The spider's image has been scraped out of the stone wall, leaving only a scar hinting at its presence at the centre of the painted web. It was, I have been variously told, picked out by a tarantata. St Paul's face, too, is largely effaced and one side wall holds the smudged outline of other figures. The paintings, according to local views in Giurdignano, go back to Byzantine times, when a monk is said to have resided in this cell and first decorated the walls.

Art historian Linda Safran, who works on the medieval Salento, however, asserts that there are no traces of Byzantine paintings here. Stylistic grounds suggest that these frescoes do not pre-date the nineteenth century. Moreover, the grotto in its present form is unlikely to be a hermit's cell, given the presence of medieval tombs immediately above.[17] Historian Gino Di Mitri (2000: 96) writes that the paintings have been redone several times, while a builder and painter from Giurdignano, whom I interviewed in 1999, confirmed that he had been commissioned to renovate these murals some thirty years ago. Apparently, it was his idea to include the tarantula in its web, although I was unable to elicit his motivation for doing so.[18] I have not been able to verify this fact through other records, but, unless found to be untrue, it suggests that the spider was brought to life here only some four decades ago.

The grotto is topped by one of the many stone monuments – of medieval origin, according to University of Lecce archaeologist Paul Arthur (2004) – dotting the Salentine landscape: a menhir, tipping slightly to one side, catching the unsuspecting eye likely to miss the excavated hollow below. Many hypotheses account for the presence of such stones widespread in the Salento: they may have served astronomical functions as ancient sundials or marked ritual sites, boundaries, crossroads or, in more mystical terms, intersecting ley lines.[19] To yet others, they designated abodes of the devil, explaining past efforts of the church to destroy and erode these stone pillars or to Christianize them through the incision of a cross. In 2006, a sign with information about the Giurdignano grotto officially marked this site as a tourist destination.

During the 1998 service, this menhir hovers above the crowd together with a loudspeaker. A table covered in white holds a Bible and religious utensils. The village priest gives his sermon and the congregation actively participates in prayers and hymns, voices mixing with the sound of birds and mopeds or tractors passing at a distance. Only this once every year did the Christian Church agree to honour a site possibly rooted in a pre-Christian past. What is more, this was to be the last time, following the decisions of Church authorities. Most of the open-air congregation is elderly and from the village of Giurdignano itself. The most senior members have taken their place at the centre of the crowd. Several black-clad women stand at the opening of the grotto at road level with their faces carved in deep and solemn wrinkles. A number of older men have positioned themselves alongside the obelisk. One leans against the ancient stone: a picture of resilience.

I recognize two or three of the younger faces; I had seen them at the chapel of Galatina that same morning. There is also Fernando. He moves around the crowd of people taking pictures from various angles. His telephoto lens stands out like the loudspeakers, time-markers in a set that could have belonged to other decades and centuries if it weren't for the clothes people are wearing and a tractor waiting to pass along the narrow road blocked by the congregation. The service concludes with the distribution of *pane benedetto*, blessed bread, traditionally made from the first grain threshed every year.[20] Then the congregation gradually flows back into town.

Some linger behind, and one last devotee arrives accompanied by her family members. She deposits a personal offering inside the cavern and bends her brow over the grotto opening until she is face to face with St Paul. Her lips move in prayer. She too has lived with the tarantula's sting, I am told by her family members. Now she has received St Paul's grace and yet, every year, she continues to pay her respects.

A year later, in June 1999, Giurdignano has a new village priest and no mass is held at this site. Just a small service consoles those for whom it holds meaning. The priest's decision, I am told by two elderly ladies who, like many of Giurdignano's inhabitants, continue to pay their respects, is based on 'higher orders' concerned about the fact that this landmark is no longer consecrated. However, even in June 2005, there are still over twenty-five candles, plant pots and flowers underneath the painted spider web.[21] Maurizio Nocera hints at another motive behind the new priest's arrangements, linked to the strong presence of (ex)tarantate at this occasion: 'He realizes that he is blessing the devil, the spider, with all those signore there.'[22]

It is unclear, however, whether anyone has danced here in honour of the tarantula and St Paul. Various elderly and young people denied this fact or said that they did not know, while researcher Luigi Chiriatti implies that this site has resounded with the beat of tambourines: 'In the night ... sounds of hides and copper-plates and cries howled at the moon, and dances, Filomena, bride of St Paul' (1996: 12). Who may have danced and for what reason remain a mystery. What is clear is that difficult-to-verify allusions abound. These are voiced not only by those who have been directly involved with the tarantula's bite, but also by researchers with or without first-hand experience of tarantism. Like travel writers in the past, those who inscribe accounts of the tarantate on paper today play a vital role in perpetuating the clash between believers and sceptics, dropping information that is at times uncontextualized, sometimes obscure because unfounded or so as not to reveal the identity of those involved, and very often cross-fertilized by hearsay. Just as St Paul's site brings to the fore tensions between believers and sceptics, an episode of Latrodectus poisoning recorded in the late 1990s, evoked heated debates for and against the tarantula.

Spider Poisoning: a Contested Case

In 1996, an actual case of spider poisoning was recorded near the town of Otranto. It brought to a peak the discourses that make up a vibrant part of what constitutes tarantism, in its curative sense, today. Five doctors from the Cardinale G. Panico Hospital of Tricase treated the young man bitten on 4 July 1996 and wrote their official report (Colonna et al. 1997: 49–50, 2000: 171–79).

The poison found its way into the body of the young male victim via a sting on the left foot. Ignored at first as an unwarranted itch, with no trace of a possible instigator, insect or thorn, ten minutes passed: the silence before the storm. Then the venom hit. Violent cramps in the left leg forced the young man's body to a halt, compelling him to take a closer look at the two lesions on his foot. Another ten minutes, and the venom fiercely contracted his stomach muscles. Others accompanied him to a first-aid centre. Analgesics helped to loosen the poison's grip, enabling the victim to be taken to the surgical unit of the Scorrano hospital. Surgery was ruled out and the intensive care unit of the Tricase hospital became the next stop in this race against the toxin. A tiny, triangular lesion, no more than three millimetres broad and marked by three holes, identified the poison's port of entry. By this stage, the venom had knotted the patient's stomach muscles and left limb into agony. Tests were administered and symptomatic therapy initiated: analgesics, muscle relaxants, antihistamines and diuretics prescribed to defy the poison. A day later, the patient was still extremely anxious, trembling, perspiring heavily and his urine had turned black. Another twenty-four hours passed before any considerable improvement was noted, recovery appeared secured, the venom on its way out, and the patient, finally, safe. A few days later, the young man was released from hospital.

From a clinical point of view, this case was resolved on the sixth day, when the patient was discharged. From an anthropological point of view, the story had only just begun. Repercussions of this bite revealed major discrepancies marking perceptions of tarantism in the contemporary Salento.[23] The medics involved confirmed that this case was exceptional in that it led to the only documentation of a contemporary case of spider poisoning based on laboratory tests available in the Salento today. However, this clinical report gives no hint of the perplexity this case caused for the medics in the intensive care unit of the Tricase hospital, or of the ethnographically specific consequences, which locate it within the Salento.

In their conversations with Luigi Chiriatti (1997b: 58–59) and myself (in March 1998), the doctors involved relate how this case presented them with a diagnostic puzzle accentuated by the following factors: firstly, the patient was suspected of snake poisoning, but the administration of an anti-viper serum had to be carefully assessed as it is not without potential allergic side effects; secondly, the location of the bite mark on the patient's left foot dispelled the hypothesis of snake poisoning, as it was unlikely that a serpent would have been able to enter the patient's boot. Moreover, the crushed shell of a snail was found inside this boot, suggesting that a smaller insect inhabiting the shell was responsible for the bite; and, thirdly, none of the doctors involved had ever come across a case of spider poisoning before, nor were they familiar with the symptoms involved.

Later enquiries among their colleagues in the Salento suggested that no instance of spider poisoning had been reported in the last fifty years or so. Initially, no link was drawn to the tarantula: it was simply one of many suspects under investigation. The patient was consulted and extensive laboratory tests were undertaken to test all possible hypotheses. Literature on spider poisoning was reviewed as the tarantula became a key suspect. Interestingly, this included De Martino's book *La terra del rimorso* (1961a), which turned out to provide essential clues: the descriptions of the tarantate's symptoms were found to correspond precisely to those of the patient. The Centro Veleni di Milano, a Milan-based unit specializing in the analysis of poisons, then tested the patient's blood sample and confirmed the tarantula's culpability.

Apparently, according to the doctors' account, the patient himself drew no links with the tarantula. Only when interviewed at a later stage did he reveal that his father and aunt had immediately suspected the spider (Chiriatti 1997b: 56). Not only his family, but also other elderly people who came to know of his case insisted that he go to Galatina. He was repeatedly warned that, if a tarantula had been responsible for the bite, he would have to dance the following year. He himself staunchly discounted tarantism as nothing but popular belief, although other members of his family had previously been bitten by the tarantula (ibid.: 56–57). Apparently, he never did dance.[24]

Media headlines, however, maximized the sensational: 'After thirty years of silence, it has struck again. The "tarantula" has returned to make its voice – and its poisonous bite – heard in the fields of the Salento' (Delle Donne 1996: 9). Moreover, a conference entitled 'Il tarantismo fra mito e realtà' (Tarantism between Myth and Reality) was organized in September 1996 to bring together researchers from both the medical and the social sciences in order to discuss this case. Links to tarantism were stressed (Chiriatti 1997b: 59): the period of recovery corresponded to the average length of tarantism rituals (three days); the bite was registered in an area identified as a mythic and elective site of the tarantula because of the relatively large number of tarantate still known to live there today; and *La terra del rimorso* (De Martino 1961a) was used as a diagnostic tool. Others criticized such correlations as reductively conflating tarantism with spider poisoning (Rivera 1996). Clearly, researchers play a key role in constructing, moulding and reinventing perceptions of tarantism today. They too may be the targets of the tarantula's modern sceptics. This scepticism was expressed with particular vehemence in another conversation I had on the very day in early August 1999 that I spoke to Francesco, who had experienced the tarantula's curse.

Tarantism as Fiction: Debates Against the Tarantula

Having finally said goodbye to Francesco and his family, my companion Bengasi, who had kindly arranged the meeting, urges me to speak to another fellow citizen: a gentleman about the age of Francesco who has been studying tarantism for many years out of personal interest. Our friend Vittorio has to leave us. I wouldn't mind leaving either, feeling more than saturated with the information from the previous interview and roasted from the heat. But it seems a chance not to be missed: an interview offered on a silver platter, so to speak, and, moreover, I sense there is another view Bengasi wants me to hear, as he has taken the trouble to arrange this second meeting without any prompting on my part. As a result, we arrive at the studio of Paolo Zacchino, a high-ceilinged space, which I recall through tired senses as a combination of office workspace and theatre prop collection. We sit facing each other on three chairs placed just inside the large, garage-like entrance opening onto the street. Paolo begins to speak in a solemn and emphatic voice:

> They have built castles in the air around tarantism. Tarantism, in our parts, is a complete invention. There is nothing that is true. It is all false.

Bengasi: There's a castle falling now, for this young lady!

Paolo: The castle must fall because ... some scholars have taken on information about tarantism always based on the view of people who were directly involved or had family members who were ... but scientifically – I will explain why, and then a scholar who has done research on this topic should answer me – the phenomenon of tarantism was born out of needs linked to the family. There may be controversies within the family. Note that almost always a teenage girl was involved. Why is it that the sting of the tarantula always affected a teenage girl? Was it because of sexual needs? Principally it was because of divergences that occurred in the families. And then the tarantula – scholars call her the dancing tarantula – is said to bite only in the summer period, during the wheat harvest, during the tobacco harvest. Now why don't the scholars explain this to me?

Let's take the example of wheat. It wasn't the women who went to reap the wheat, it was the older people and they were the ones to have direct contact with the grain, but note that these elderly people were never bitten. First, as to the tobacco harvest, entire families were involved in harvesting. But why did the tarantula bite only the young women? Did this tarantula have a sixth sense and go in search of a particular hand or a particular foot of a young woman to bite? There has been a lot of speculation about tarantism. And then, the other aspect is that tarantism is spoken about only with regard to Nardò and Galatina. Why doesn't anyone speak about Galatone, Copertino, Leverano, Veglie, Salice?[25]

Bengasi: In past years, Copertino was also spoken about.

Paolo: Well, okay, but always marginally.

93

Karen: Also the area of Otranto is often mentioned.

Paolo: Yes, because the phenomenon then spread out, the affair assumed county-wide dimensions; but beyond these towns? Even in the area of Brindisi, wheat is grown and tobacco, etc., but these phenomena don't exist. So I am convinced, very convinced – and scholars will have to demonstrate otherwise – about the family issue. And nobody knows how it was born. How were the various traditions born? Something happened and then assumed larger dimensions.

Karen: Often there was no real bite, often the tarantata wasn't actually bitten by a spider.

Paolo: No, the tarantula has nothing to do with it. It may be an illness relieved through music. It may be a need ... Today, if someone has convulsions, etc., there is the hospital. But, yesterday, when they had these moments of illness, these things ... well, what do you say, has she been bitten by the tarantula? Let's see ... I took part at one of these dances of a tarantata and am still left with the impression of pretence. It was behind my house and complete pretence. This person danced for an hour, for half an hour, etc.; people came and threw one hundred lire or two hundred lire[26] onto the blanket, and when they finished playing and she was tired – it's logical that after dancing she was tired – maybe she's calmed herself, maybe she's healed; and when the people have gone away she collects all of the money and puts it away.

Karen: But why pretend to suffer to make money?

Paolo: To make money or to convince a parent who didn't want to give their daughter in marriage to Tizio, Caio, Sempronio,[27] to convince the parents that her cure could be a husband, so this one danced until her mother said: 'Let's go to St Paul, it's necessary to go to Galatina, for this young girl a husband is needed,' and so they were convinced.

Bengasi: It's important to look at the customs of the families, how it was possible to use this phenomenon for personal means. It's important now to go from one part to the other and to see how they coincide. I think it's necessary to reconcile everything: I don't believe ... I believe ... like you hear about Padre Pio, who performs lots of miracles.[28]

Paolo: I take many situations into careful consideration and these lead me to not believe.

Bengasi: The Church doesn't believe in these miracles.

Karen: But what about the tarantate who jump up onto the altar, even though they entered the chapel without strength, carried in the arms of others?

Paolo: In a word, a young woman! Wouldn't you manage to jump onto the altar?

Karen: But also the old people ...

94

Paolo: No, there weren't any old people. There were some women who reached the age of forty, but they are the kind of women who put themselves in front of a cart and pull it for you. To jump onto the altar ... for a young woman who is emancipated, isn't difficult. It's just like with the unlikely story of when they pass through the chairs ... So what happened with the phenomenon of the chairs? There was someone who, as there was a chair on the ground, slipped through it. Contorting themselves they could pass underneath, and then the others recounted: 'Madonna! She passed through the chair!' But it's not true that she passed through it. It's not possible. It's absurd. But word spread, that she passed through the chair ... They also came to interview me, those from the RAI, but then I was disappointed that they didn't take my view into account.

Bengasi: They help themselves to create spectacles, broadcasting any kind of rubbish.

Paolo: Then they spit on what you say ... what you hear, you should say! It's not like you always find what you want ... Now I don't know what your research is aimed at, but I would study all of this more thoroughly, but scientifically and not by hearsay, because there is lots of hearsay. If you interview a person who has been directly involved they can't say: 'No, it's not true!' having already been involved in interviews, in newspapers. They tell you: 'Yes, it's true! I've been miraculously healed. I went to Galatina, to St Paul, I went through this or that, etc.' They will most definitely tell you this, if there still are any. But, most definitely, there will also be people who know the life of the family, the various reasons, and so you need to make this comparison: in other words, this one is telling me this in one way, and this one in another way ...

When I went to Galatina, I was participating in theatre shows. What I saw in Galatina were theatrical acts, there was nothing true, all this movement that they did, all these scenes, you saw a normal person, tired, that shows immediately, but that's it, there's no illness, no bite, nothing; it's all pretence, it's all staged, it's all a show ... they were up to all sorts of mischief; as you said, they climbed onto the altar ... now it's all forbidden, but you saw those who climbed onto the altar, and it's not like the one who didn't manage to walk climbed up. The young girls climbed up, the young women, etc., who had, perhaps, even rehearsed at home, climbing onto a table or a bench!

As my companion Bengasi and I drive away, having said goodbye to Paolo, I can't help but feel as if I had just walked out of a classroom. Paolo had made every effort to debunk all myths and miracles associated with the tarantula. He had reiterated various points De

Martino isolated as proof against any direct cause-and-effect link between the actual threat of spider poisoning and the crises of the tarantate. However, whereas De Martino interpreted these facts as culturally specific responses to suffering, Paolo dismissed everything as pretence. His view highlights the potential power play and manipulation for personal means that may underlie cases of tarantism, but his stance also entails the risk of rejecting this entire phenomenon on the basis of its symptoms (dispelled as inventions).

However, a look at others' sceptical responses shows how the notion of invention comes into play to varying degrees for both believers and sceptics.[29] Some of the elderly farming community in the Salento continue to equate tarantism with spider poisoning. 'The soil has become cold because of the pesticides, which have killed all the spiders. That is why there are no longer any tarantate,' one elderly farmer told me. The (apparent?) eradication of the spider provides a straightforward explanation for the extinction of tarantism. For many, tarantism is a cause of amusement or embarrassment. 'Today we laugh about it!' For some, tarantism was never more than a fable. 'Ah, the tarantate – but that's a legend – I don't believe in them!' A few, moreover, do not know about tarantism. The subject was taboo in some families. A young female student at the University of Lecce confirmed that she had never heard about tarantism until it was discussed in a university course she attended.

For others belief in tarantism is irreconcilable with Christian or biomedical logic. On the morning of St Paul's festival, I spoke at length with a newspaper vendor in Galatina: 'I don't believe in it', he argued, 'because I follow the Church. The Church and medicine don't admit these things.' This point was also brought home to me during a conversation with a middle-aged woman in a small town near Tricase: 'Tarantism is a thing of the devil ... The only doctor is our Lord!' For some, tarantism may have had its validity in the past, but is clearly outdated today, as Antonio Antonacci (1988: 1), a priest from Galatina, stresses:

> As regards the problem of the 'tarantate,' there are people who have remained fixated, like a broken clock, in a remote past ... Tarantolism is a distant reminiscence. And, it is known that people also want to see themselves in this 'reminiscence,' as if to project themselves with gratification into a past of fears and difficulties ... the subtle denigration of the South, also in this field, is inexhaustible.

When asked to speak about this phenomenon for the purposes of my research, Antonacci explained his unwillingness to do so on the basis of the fact that he considered tarantism to have been a falsehood.

A retired secondary-school teacher and relative of a deceased tarantata, meanwhile, argues that the violent and traumatic roots of tarantism leave the afflicted without trust or self-esteem and with feelings of not being worthy of joy or pleasure, leading to vicious cycles of suffering, which could have been avoided with psychiatric and pharmaceutical treatment: 'It's a form of self-punishment. The afflicted punish themselves by excluding themselves, because they feel excluded. This leads to a vicious circle, because this behaviour of self-exclusion easily becomes a source of embarrassment for others, who then begin to deliberately exclude these individuals too.' Yet others point to the conceptual changes modern health care has brought with it. A psychologist at a psychiatric centre in Lecce expands on this: 'In the past, someone was either mad or a tarantata. The concepts of depression, burnout or nervous breakdown didn't exist. All were classified as "mad". The diversification of medical concepts has contributed to the end of tarantism.' Music therapist Rita Cappello, meanwhile, adds: 'It is very likely that symptoms of tarantism persist today under a new name, but using tarantism today instead of music therapy would be like teaching a child to learn to count on its fingers without ever giving it access to a computer.'

Diverging views coexist in the Salento today, revealing various levels of belief in the historical validity or reality of tarantism. It is widely dismissed as invention or fiction, providing good reasons not to link symptoms of tarantism to contemporary disturbances. And yet the views voiced by health-care practitioners suggest that although the tarantate may no longer exist their symptoms persist, cloaked in new terminology. The tarantula spider may have been eradicated from Salentine soil and the beliefs of its younger generations, but experiences of affliction comparable to those of the tarantate have not been eradicated with an equally reassuring certainty. Show business, as the next chapter reveals, helps to distract attention from this fact, nominating the tarantula, instead, first and foremost as an emblem of local identity.

Notes

1. These are the words of a speaker at a conference on tarantism held during the days leading up to the festivities of St Peter and Paul.

2. On my return to the Salento in 2001, I am told that Francesco, too, has passed away. I record this interview here in his memory.

3. It remains unclear when exactly Francesco's afflictions began and how long they lasted: he speaks of both twenty and thirty years ago, while his wife cites 1967 as the year of his last major crisis.

4. Francesco uses the word *abbandonato* here, which may be variously translated as abandoned, marooned, forsaken, uncared-for, helpless or forlorn.

5. The Italian term *quintale* refers to the metric equivalent of approximately 100 kg.

6. Francesco uses various terms to refer to the symptoms of his crises: *male* (translated here as affliction, although it has broader connotations of evil, ill, wrong, misfortune, adversity, trouble, as well as illness, disease, pain or ache); *guasto* (damage, breakdown or failure); and *malattia* (illness, malady, infirmity or ailment).

7. The Italian name *organetto,* used by Francesco, refers to the diatonic or button accordion found in central and southern Italy.

8. One hundred thousand lire is the approximate equivalent of 50 euros (using the conversion rate of 1,936.27 lire to one euro from 1 January 2002, when the euro was first introduced).

9. Francesco uses the Italian term *scherzi* (jokes, jests, pranks or tricks) to refer to the behaviour of the tarantate at Galatina.

10. Francesco refers here to a phenomenon widely associated with the tarantate and generally viewed as inexplicable by those who believed.

11. Here I pick up the term 'shadow' used by Francesco earlier to describe the presence of St Paul.

12. RAI is the Italian broadcasting service, Radio Televisione Italiana.

13. Lecce, 2 February 1998.

14. Nocera refers here to the film by Miscuglio et al. (1981).

15. Lecce, 1 April 2006.

16. Brindisi, 15 November 1997, and Lecce, 10 June 1998.

17. Personal communication, 6 February 2006.

18. Giurdignano, 18 August 1999.

19. Leylines are said to connect strategic geographical points such as megaliths or ancient monuments. These alignments are associated with magnetic or magical forces by some and dismissed as pseudoscience by others.

20. The group Mascarimirì sings about this in their song 'Pizzica RAÏ' on their album *Triciu* (Romano 2006): 'Santu Paulu de Giurdignanu con il primo pane tra la mano' (St Paul of Giurdignano with the first bread in his hand).
21. I thank Linda Safran for providing me with photos of the grotto from this year.
22. Galatina, 28 June 1999.
23. For a collection of interviews on this case see Chiriatti (1997b: 45–84).
24. Giorgio Di Lecce, Lecce, 23 October 1998, confirmed this after speaking to the young man two years later.
25. The towns listed belong to an area south-west and west of Lecce [see Fig. 0.2].
26. One hundred lire would be approximately 5 cents (using the conversion rate of 1,936.27 lire to one euro from 1 January 2002, when the euro was first introduced).
27. Italian equivalent of Tom, Dick and Harry, referring to any ordinary person.
28. Padre Pio (1887–1968) of San Giovanni Rotondo, Apulia, whose icons, statues and devotees are widespread in Apulia, was sanctified on 16 June 2002.
29. These views are taken from field notes based on interviews in various towns throughout the Salento written in the period from June 1997 to August 1999.

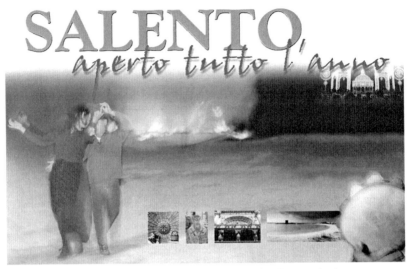

Fig. 4.1 Salento 'Open All Year Round', 2001 (postcard: Azienda di Promozione Turistica di Lecce, Martano Editrice and Radici di Pietra; photo: Fernando Bevilacqua; claim: Nello Wrona).

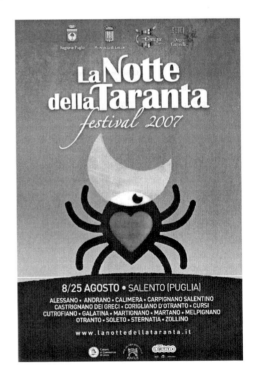

Fig. 4.2 Poster of 'La Notte della Taranta', August 2007 (© Istituto Diego Carpitella).

100

Chapter 4
Ads and Antidotes:
Celebrity versus Conservation

> Down in the Salento we have the sun and the beautiful sea
> and with the tambourine people dance and play,
> but this 'ethnic music' has become like a postcard
> of a fake Salento of nights and tarantulas.
> I am 'ethnic' but infuriated because the tambourine
> mustn't become like a ring through the nose.
> Applaud the politicians,
> who invent the festivals and so everything seems to go well.
> And so I say: Heavy blows with sounds and songs,
> Heavy blows for all and without mercy.
> I am an infuriated 'ethnic' and one thing I have to say,
> If we don't speak now, tell me when we should speak.[1]
>
> Roberto Raheli, Album *Mazzate Pesanti*, 2004

The group Aramirè takes a verbally militant approach, as the lyrics of their song 'Mazzate Pesanti' (Heavy Blows), performed to the pizzica's beats, shows. Roberto Raheli, director of the group and author of this song, speaks out strongly against the commercialization and exploitation of the music, dance and territory of the Salento. The inside cover photo of this album shows an equally evocative and all too common scene in the Salento: a rubbish dump of abandoned washing machines, stoves and fridges on the outskirts of a village marked by a flag post sign reading 'Divieto di scarico' (No Waste Dumping). A ban acting as a magnet. Raheli spotlights further contradictions:

For me discourses need to be more complete, regarding the Salento as a whole without isolating questions of music and dance. It's no good attracting tourists to festivals and other events if the beaches remain dirty. It's no good speaking of diversifying events throughout the seasons if then all major events are programmed in August. It's no good spending heaps of money on mega-concerts if the traditional stone walls all around the Salento are falling down.[2]

The tarantula's music and dance have become a free-for-all device, abounding in inconsistencies and bringing to the fore key issues – questions of authenticity, invented traditions and identity, in particular – associated with the so-called 'revival' or revitalization of musical traditions more generally (Hobsbawn and Ranger 1983; Grenier and Guilbault 1990; Livingston 1999; Sant Cassia 2000). This is not without friction, as Paolo Apolito (2000), lecturer in social anthropology at the University of Salerno, brilliantly discusses. Whereas only a decade or two ago tarantism was a source of shame, fostering conceptions of Salentines and Apulians as poor and ignorant, this has been reversed today. 'This time it is the Apulians, in particular a cultural group, which is urbanized, critical and post-modern, who claim tarantism as a positive, noble and profound sign of their history and identity' (ibid.: 139). Surfing this wave, De Martino's book *La terra del rimorso* (1961a) 'often not read and not understood, has become a strong source of interest, concentrated, just like an emblem, a banner, of local identity' (Apolito 2000: 139).

In this context, the tarantula has become 'a symbol that stands for itself' (Wagner 1986), with a certain autonomy in relation to its users, showing how the invention of meaning involves an unrelenting process of transformation. Whereas in the past the tarantula's ritual was part of a cultural complex deeply rooted within everyday life, these links were cleanly cut by the 1990s, and tarantism appears to be no more and no less than a free-floating spot or slogan, as aptly labelled by Apolito (2000: 141): 'Tarantism is not an essence which is in some way configurable and identifiable. Instead it involves all that can be said about it.' As a manifold tool, applicable to multiple purposes, the tarantula is as ubiquitous as ever.

A look at four specific initiatives that have brought the spider back to fame, locally, nationally and internationally, illustrates this. First, experimental techno-pizzica jam sessions provide examples of attempts by intellectuals and musicians to adapt the tarantula's music and dance to contemporary music trends. The festival of San Rocco presents a second key initiative and a mecca for pizzica fans from all over the Salento, Apulia, Italy and elsewhere, vibrating to the pizzica's rhythms from dusk to dawn on the night of 15 August each year. Thirdly, the annual 'Night of the Tarantula' concert held in August has become the diva of summer celebrations, taking the spider on tour worldwide. Finally, this large-scale event is offset by a low-key local initiative, La Sagra dei Curli, the Festival of the Spinning Top, representative of less formal, more intimate get-togethers. The pizzica's beat is the dynamo behind all of these occasions.

Taranta-muffin, Techno-pizzica, Tarantavirus: Hybridizing the Pizzica

One heated, omnipresent discourse regards the contamination of Salentine music. Some deliberately incite processes of hybridization whereas others seek to record and reproduce 'the old ways' as much as possible. French academic Georges Lapassade (1994) is among those with an active interest in so-called hybrid musical forms and their relation to discourses on identity.

Lapassade has suggested that musicians such as those of the Salentine rap group Sud Sound System can be defined as today's tarantati. This group coined the term 'taranta-muffin' to refer to a mix of Jamaican reggae and their own musical heritage, knitting together rhythms with 'local' and 'global' connections, integrating the 'foreign' and 'familiar'. Where musical creativity reaches out to engulf influences from elsewhere, Lapassade has drawn historical connections to stress that contemporary performances of the pizzica provide essential symbols of group identity and a key to Salentine culture as such.

With this in mind, Lapassade lists potential points of contact between the performances by the Sud Sound System and the rituals of the tarantate: first, in line with traditional tarantism songs, the young rap group insists on using the *Leccese* dialect, emphasizing its territorial origins. Second, this group's concerts may be viewed as ritualistic on the basis of the extensive involvement of the audience. A 'rotating microphone' may mark these occasions. It is passed between performers and spectators, allowing participants to contribute improvised lines. Third, certain pieces by the Sud Sound System, such as 'Afro ragga taranta jazz' on the LP *Comu na Petra* (1996), explicitly contain pizzica rhythms. These connections cannot, however, make up for the deep

103

discrepancies between historical rituals of tarantism and contemporary performances of the Sud Sound System. Interestingly, the musicians themselves initially opposed being categorized as *nuovi* or new tarantati, objecting to associations with a cult weighed down with prejudices, but subsequently, with the new pizzica craze, began to promote this image themselves.

Meanwhile, academics Lapassade and Piero Fumarola actively promoted other experiments of 'contaminating' traditional Salentine music, including the techno-pizzica (Maggiorelli 1996).[3] During the 1997 Venice carnival, to which a number of Salentine groups were invited, an initial 'jam session' was organized with the Sud Sound System and Gli Ucci, a group of *anziani* (elderly) well respected for their musical skills and renditions of the tarantula's music in its 'traditional' sense (Durante 2005: 60–61). Since then, similar events in Lecce and elsewhere have explored the potential of this musical cocktail. Daniele Durante (1999: 174) draws attention to similarities between past rituals and such techno-pizzica events:

> Whoever enters this musical atmosphere loses control of inhibitory restraints and looks to the music as a vector to reach 'other' dimensions in which to forget, discharge, digest or eliminate the poisons and tensions of daily life ... To interrupt this sonorous flow almost brings about a physical unease in the dancers, comparable to that of the tarantate at one time, and to ravers today ... A further analogy with the therapeutic orchestra is represented in the pursuit of the instrumentalists to excite[4] the tarantula by taking turns in approaching the ear of the tarantata with their instruments. In our case, this was possible through the use of the microphone. Taking turns to distance ourselves or come close both with the tambourine and with our voices, we had the impression of penetrating the bodies of the dancers. Many dancers, in fact, placed themselves close to the loudspeakers, knowing well that, when very strong sound waves are emitted, it is no longer the ear that hears, but the body.

Inevitably, such comparisons require careful and critical consideration. However, although the techno-pizzica has been scorned by some, it is a good example of how the active and deliberate involvement of intellectuals in the promotion of research linked to the tarantula's music and dance is fundamental to contemporary discourses on tarantism.[5]

The 1970s saw initial attempts, led by young intellectuals and musicians, at recording the traditional music of the Salento as performed by elderly members of society. Often these endeavours met with resistance, as they evoked memories of a past tinged with suffering and anguish, often looked back on with embarrassment. Many did not want to remember (Chiriatti 1998). Despite the ardent efforts of a few passionate individuals, it was not until the 1990s that Salentine music took off in grand style. By the year 2000, some fifty groups had sprouted out of the ground, while more established groups, with success in Italy and elsewhere, numbered a dozen or so.[6]

Dance ethnologist Giuseppe Gala (2002b: 48) identifies the reasons for the pizzica's boom in the 1990s not only in intrinsic factors (the impacts of the spider's seductive myth and the tambourine's rhythmic repetition) but also in external ones, including choices other than drug addiction; research and cinematography on tarantism; the fashion of world music and 'ethnic things'; the influence of esoteric, New Age philosophies and of popular figures in the Italian popular music scene (such as Eugenio Bennato, Teresa De Sio, Daniele Sepe and the group Nuova Compagnia di Canto Popolare), as well as generational fashions more generally. A member of the discussion forum on the website www.pizzicata.it takes up this point:

> The success of the pizzica is certainly in part a fashionable and commercial phenomenon, but in my opinion it also represents a response to globalization, currently wanting to force us all to listen to the same music, to eat the same things (perhaps at McDonald's), to think in the same way, not to speak of war. With the recovery of popular music, traditions and local identities in general, many are looking for a way to fill a vacuum of values they feel inside… This is a phenomenon that is happening in the whole world and it is positive if it doesn't lead to the construction of new fences: a community can have a strong identity but it is important that it is a community that is open to the outside … after all, many of our traditions were born from a mixture of cultures that have influenced our land.[7]

Similarly, the late Giorgio Di Lecce, director of the group Arakne Mediterranea and lecturer in the history of dance at the University of Lecce, explained: 'In my opinion, it is because a generation has passed. Those of today no longer have points of reference as the generation before did. The young people today are in need of roots. They are looking for points of reference.'[8] The notion of *terra*, of earth or native land (translated here in the sense of roots or origins), is evoked to speak about a lack of coordinates in everyday life. Di Lecce takes up a common discourse associating modernity with the challenges and hardships of being 'rootless', despite the incomparably improved socio-economic conditions of younger generations in comparison with their predecessors.

The pizzica's burst of popularity has also created a source of intense rivalry and back-stabbing regarding questions of origins, musical execution and ownership. Many insist on having been the first to revitalize this music, claiming their right to others' acknowledgement, if not to copyrights. Rather than considering the efforts of various individuals and groups in creating the momentum and popularity that the pizzica currently enjoys, energy, words, time and money are, often indirectly, invested in fighting for 'first place' – despite equally insistent claims regarding the ancient and medieval precedents of this music and dance. Depending on the perspective taken, various names are pinpointed as key catalysts behind the pizzica's recent revitalization, although overall it is probably fair to say that momentum picked up over the years through the engagement and dedication of the many who spurred on this movement through both enthusiasm and competition.[9]

In 2007, the CD *Tarantavirus* was brought out in conjunction with the events calendar *quiSalento*, presenting the combined musical talents of two Salentine stars: Uccio Aloisi, retired farmer in his eighties and charismatic singer and tambourine player of the group Gli Ucci (Raheli et al. 2004), and Cesare dell'Anna, talented trumpet player in his forties, known for his performances inspired by Balkan music. '"Tarantavirus – the impoverished spider" is a disc of passage, from the ancient to the modern, from the "old" to the young, it is a representation of the meridian spirit through a "technological" lens, a natural "contamination" of ancient instigations with new technologies, new desires and new dances' (Anon. 2007: 81).[10] *Tarantavirus* is one of hundreds of CDs on the burgeoning market of the tarantula's music and dance. Efforts to revitalize this music and dance, of which the Festival of San Rocco is a key example, have become inextricably intertwined with their commercialization.

The Festival of San Rocco: Revitalizing and Commercializing Traditions

I still remember as if it was yesterday that incredible shove he gave me, perhaps with the elbow, which pushed me into the centre of the circle; I raise my eyes, and find myself face to face with a gypsy; he is large with dark skin and his fiery eyes are fixed on me; his body moves lightly in spite of its massive structure ... wake up! phew ... with incredible potency he skims my face ... with no time to reflect, I dodge; my adrenaline rises to never imagined levels, I'm afraid, my eyes search for my preceptor; he plays, his squinting eyes focused on nothing; careful! ... blow after violent blow follows; there's no time to think or to be afraid; I let myself go ... I dance. (Probo 1996)

With these words Lamberto Probo, member of the group Officina Zoë, describes how, for the first time, he finds himself dancing the scherma. An old man and teacher had propelled him into this situation. The occasion is 15 August, the festival of San Rocco, and the venue Torrepaduli, a small town in the south-western cape: the most well-known 'fortress' of the scherma today (Di Lecce 1992; Melchioni 1999; Tarantino 2001; Chiriatti and Miscuglio 2004; Monaco 2006; Inguscio 2007). Until the first mass on 16 August tambourine players of all ages enact their modern-day vigil (Torsello 1997b), singing and beating their instruments, standing in tight circles of performers, opening and closing spontaneously, within which the pizzica pizzica and scherma are danced.[11]

At Torrepaduli, nowadays, courtship and duels go hand in hand, but it was not always like this. These crowds are recent and, apparently, this festival's popularity among performers goes back no more than two decades. Prior to the 1980s, 'the festival of St Rocco in Torrepaduli was', as Giovanni Pellegrino (1995) writes, 'the last shore on which tambourine players performed, or rather "resisted": those last players were almost all very old and resigned. This age-old festival had become reduced to a pigtail, which wore out shortly after midnight.' The resurrection of this festival, paralleling similar endeavours throughout Europe, was part of more widespread attempts to revitalize traditional Salentine celebrations eroded in the post-war period, in the face of social fractures left by large-scale emigration and the advent of everything that stood for modernization (Boissevain 1992; Tak 2000).

In 1982, a group of Salentines decided to promote *il ritorno a San Rocco,* the return to St Rocco. They sought out musicians and dancers to find out what factors brought them to San Rocco or kept them away; approached cultural and academic institutions, as well as local authorities to seek advice and support for this event; and relaunched the tambourine, as an emblem of past forms of socializing, at the Festa del Tamburello, the Festival of the Tambourine, in Cutrofiano eight days prior to 15 August, to publicize and warm up for San Rocco. In subsequent years, slowly but steadily, the tambourine made its way into the limelight and the festival of Torrepaduli has now become a major focus for celebrations of Italy's national holiday, *ferragosto*.[12]

In 2005, I arrive at Torrepaduli at 2 a.m. and there is a two-kilometre queue of cars leading up to the village. The town centre and piazza in front of San Rocco's sanctuary are packed. We need to take care not to step on dogs or people sitting on the litter-covered ground. The atmosphere is heavy with drained, dreadlocked bodies, many appearing stoned, sprawled on the ground: although marginal in number these young people, generally labelled as *punkabbestia* for their unkempt looks and ragged pet dogs, stand out in an area where locals dress up for the occasion and the average person would rarely be seen sitting on the curb of the road.[13] It is hard to ignore the sense of chaos and disregard that permeates the air, although excessive drunkenness or aggression is absent. On the main piazza circles of musicians hold back throngs of onlookers and carve out spaces in which dancers move. These circles form spontaneously, with participants joining in and dropping out, determining whether circles last or simply dissolve. Some continue for hours, with spectators containing and animating the performances, and create a stark contrast to the confusion elsewhere around the festival. Where rules are respected, seduction and playful competition reign.

Despite this success in attracting crowds today, many of those who never deserted this festival and worked to revitalize it are unhappy about the current situation. 'It's nothing but chaos' is the most common criticism, initiating fiery discussions between traditionalists and modernists (Metafune 2002). Giovanni Pellegrino (2002) draws up a balance sheet twenty years after the initial return to San Rocco, isolating two main problems: the 'acoustic pollution' of market stalls, with loudspeakers booming over the sound of the tambourines played live, and the increasing presence of 'invasive' drums and African rhythms. 'With every respect for other cultures and their fans,' Pellegrino (2002) appeases his readers, 'I believe ... that we're speaking about the most classical meeting of Salentine tambourines and the rhythms of the pizzica and of nothing else.'

By 2005, leaflets of the manifesto *Proteggiamo Torrepaduli*, Let's Protect Torrepaduli, aimed at safeguarding this festival, present four clear demands: respect for the devotees of San Rocco; a zone in front of St Rocco's sanctuary reserved for 'traditional circles' without drums; no participation in circles by absolute beginners; and, no more than one couple appearing in a circle at one time.[14] The subtitle, 'Awareness Campaign for the Recovery and Protection of One of the Last Traditional Salentine Festivals', raises questions about how traditional a revitalized festival can be and, more importantly, what purposes its apparent traditional qualities may serve. Where continuity is ruptured, as Hobsbawn (1983: 13) points out, reference to the past often disguises other motives, hidden agendas, 'exercises in social engineering', if not overt discrimination. Commercial factors are often the first to be highlighted, as the pizzica with its mystical roots in the Salento has helped place this area in a prime position on European tourist maps.

Although widespread efforts have sought to make the tarantula's music and dance accessible on a large scale at the Festival of San Rocco, these endeavours increasingly clash with accusations of and interests in commercialization. Desires to make this festival appealing to everyone are questioned, as certain participants, such as the punkabbestia, challenge social norms and expectations. Despite calls for the traditional and authentic, San Rocco presents fertile soil for the invention of tradition, as women dance the scherma and the pizzica is danced to African drums. As these drums are marginalized and the tambourine prioritized, notions of 'contamination' or 'hybridization' are once again defied. These tensions equally mark the mega-concert of the Night of the Tarantula, the spider's first and foremost spot [see Fig. 4.2].

La Notte della Taranta: a Music and Media Spectacle

On 27 August 2005, by 10 p.m. the eighth edition of La Notte della Taranta, the Night of the Tarantula, is in full swing.[15] Some have nicknamed it *la notte fatale*, the fatal night (Santoro 2005b). I have just arrived at Melpignano, having skirted the long queue of cars waiting to turn off the Lecce-Maglie motorway to find a parking spot, on a friend's motorbike. The well-loved elderly singer Uccio Aloisi and his band are up on stage, their faces projected onto various screens suspended from the ex-cloister walls next to the grand stage, surrounded by an estimated throng of some eighty thousand listeners (Maruccio 2005). The atmosphere is lively and light-hearted. This is obviously the place to be if you want to listen to Salentine music in concert grandeur, enjoy a warm summer night get-together or care to be seen where the action is. Street vendors selling food and 'ethnic' jewellery make the most of this night. Wine, T-shirts and shoes with the spider logo of this 2005 version are also on sale: a first-time marketing stunt to promote local products in tandem with this occasion (Anon. 2005). People dance, chat and hang out, packed like sardines closer to the stage, and standing or sitting in more dispersed groups on the edges.

Backstage, meanwhile, there are snacks and drinks for free for those who have the status or connections for an entry pass. A large number of the Salento's current centre-left government, including its president Giovanni Pellegrino, are here. Other significant politicians have not missed this occasion either. Among them are Massimo D'Alema, leader of the national party Democratici di Sinistra, as well as Nichi Vendola, member of the left-wing party Rifondazione Comunista and current president of the region of Apulia. On stage, well-known Italian stars – Francesco De Gregori, Giovanna Marini, Piero Pelù and Sonia Bergamasco, to name some of the most famous – take turns behind the microphone with Salentine performers: seventy singers and musicians making up the Orchestra Popolare la Notte della Taranta, directed by Ambrogio Sparagna, doing this job for a second year round. Newspapers, meanwhile, have announced the participation of a Chinese television troupe (Presicce 2005), as well as initiatives towards inserting this night into the *Enciclopedia Italiana Treccani* (Indennitate 2005; Vendola 2005). The spider is back in action, many times magnified by the media, and thousands are dancing to its tune.

This highly controversial jewel of Salentine cultural policymakers was inaugurated in 1998. On the evening of 24 August 1998, eleven Salentine music groups performed their musical repertoires in nine different villages of the Grecìa Salentina, a region south of the Salentine capital of Lecce, in which *Griko* or Greek dialects are still spoken by a small minority.[16] By 11.30 p.m., musicians and spectators converged on the centrally located town of Melpignano, where a final concert including all participants was staged. This spectacle had been rehearsed for three days preceding the event under the direction of Neapolitan musician Daniele Sepe. Crowds in the hundreds tightly packed the main town square, where a large stage was floodlit in bright colours. Performers of all ages sang, danced and played in an as yet unprecedented collaborative effort. The crowd participated frenetically.

Circles of tambourine players and dancers formed, broke up and re-formed below the stage amidst a flash of cameras and enthusiastic applause, until the concert was officially concluded with an announcement by Maurizio Agamennone, ethnomusicologist on the scientific committee of this event: 'See you all at the Night of the Tarantula '99!' His invite signalled the pizzica's step into the limelight of what has become a major annual festival within the world music scene.[17]

From the very beginning, controversies – both among the musicians themselves and with respect to the 'outsiders' involved, such as the Neapolitan musical director and two university professors with major organizational responsibilities – brought to the forefront notions of identity played out on stage. Promoted by the Istituto Diego Carpitella, inaugurated in 1998 to document and encourage research on local traditions (Santoro 2005a: 93), this night, bringing together so many of the Salento's pizzica enthusiasts, was for many a great success. For others, the pleasure evoked did not outweigh underlying dilemmas.

A heated debate about the link between tradition and modernity in Salentine music emerged in the local papers subsequent to the first occasion.[18] Opinions appeared to be divided into two main camps. One side spoke of the need for an active confrontation of the Salento's musicians with other types of music, in order to elaborate the existing repertoire of Salentine music through 'hybridization' or 'contamination' with other styles (labelled ethnic, techno, New Age, etc.), thereby fostering innovation and diversity in a context within which 'the same songs are continually fried and refried' (V. Santoro 2001). The other side argued that any kind of popular music was inherently subject to a process of 'natural' change, but nevertheless staunchly underlined the importance of not forcing this process. Whereas it was seen as inevitable that certain groups were, for instance, influenced by Balkan music, considering the strong influx of people from these regions to southern Italy in recent years, intellectually imposed projects 'conceived at a table' (Raheli 1998) were strongly disputed.

As in its first year on stage, this event continues to attract enormous crowds, as well as immense criticism. 'The syndrome of the tarantula', Gino Di Mitri (2001) writes, 'is transversal, invasive as an enticing pest: it pleases the anti-global supporters of a home-made "buena vista social forum" just as much as right-wing municipalities engaged in (why not?) the popularistic road to tarantism.' In fact, performances of *musica popolare* such as the pizzica have accompanied the electoral campaigns of both right- and left-wing political candidates over the years. Generally speaking, however, initial inputs leading to the re-appropriation of tarantism and its music are intrinsically related to a left-wing political ideology – still considered the most politically correct in the pizzica milieu – focused on promoting and defending popular culture and local traditions.

Significantly, problems that have shaken up the organization of the Notte della Taranta and the very foundations of the Istituto Carpitella are linked not only to divergent opinions among the scientific and artistic committee, but also to the interests of politicians engaged in this event. As Gino Di Mitri (2001) states: 'What's the target? Visibility in the media, popularity among the pizzica aficionados, publicity and votes!' Technology and visibility have become major priorities, as has the creation of a Night of the Tarantula Foundation aimed at promoting research and performances in the field of popular music through a permanent Night of the Tarantula Orchestra (Torsello 2007). Further discussions regard the institutionalization and legislation of popular music and archiving resources (V. Santoro 2005b). Moreover, whereas initially criticisms were voiced about the vast discrepancies in local government expenditure for cultural programmes focused on 'cultivated' rather than 'popular' music, the pizzica has now become a major market label.

In the summer of 2003, ex-drummer of the group Police Stewart Copeland was in charge of the Orchestra Popolare la Notte della Taranta, taking it on its first European tour in the summer of 2004, including the capital cities of Athens, Brussels, Paris and Rome. In February 2006, the Venice Carnival concluded with a smaller edition of this show (Barone 2006). Two months later, local and national newspapers hailed the orchestra's Beijing concert, with fifty thousand paying fans, as a unique promotion for Italy at large (Presicce 2006).[19] 'For once, I am really proud of my homeland,' says one enthusiast.[20] For others, it is an occasion of yet further disillusionment. 'I am deeply ashamed and fear that the degradation of this *vicenda*, this initiative, has arrived at a point of no return.'[21] Critics add that the money used for this event could have promoted vast local initiatives, while politicians and cultural managers plan the next stops for the Night of the Tarantula musicians: Jordan and the Football World Cup Championships in Germany (Indennitate 2006).

In 2007, the Night of the Tarantula celebrated its tenth anniversary with a focus on integrating other music traditions from the Mediterranean basin, promoting female voices and celebrating related Apulian traditions (Quarta 2007a). Prior to the grand night, two weeks of concerts brought various Salentine music groups on stage in fifteen municipalities of the Grecìa Salentina, as well as the towns of Otranto and Andrano (Quarta 2007b: 77).

La Notte della Taranta has, in many ways, come to epitomize the contemporary revitalization of the pizzica.[22] Warnings abound. 'Dance and sing,' writes Dinko Fabris (2005) in the national newspaper *La Repubblica*, 'but, please, leave the poor tarantulas be, who, besides, should be a protected species.' Roberto Raheli is more adamant: 'The Night of the Tarantula arrives in the very delicate context of the re-appropriation of almost lost songs, like an elephant in a crystal factory.'[23] While this event has become by far the most extravagant and publicized concert of the tarantula's music and dance, there are some who have always boycotted it, making their act of absence a statement in itself.

Meanwhile, a snapshot of another summer night in 1998, the year the Night of the Tarantula was first staged, provides a glimpse of another festivity, much more intimate and small-scale, within which the tarantula surfaces both through its music and, what is more, through the improvised re-enactment of elements of the tarantate's rituals by one of the female participants, Tanya Pagliara, who explicitly declares herself to be a (modern) tarantata.

La Sagra dei Curli: a Community Festival

'Do only that which enchants you,' the late Antonio Verri, much-loved Salentine poet and writer, had said. La Sagra dei Curli, the Festival of the Spinning Top, is dedicated to his memory and to this endeavour.[24]

It is 1 August 1998, a Saturday in Vignacastrisi, a small town south of Otranto. I arrive with Tanya, in her early thirties, whom I had met in a sociology of religions class at the University of Lecce. She is an artist and two of her recent exhibitions revolved around the tarantula. Last summer, she and others sought out abandoned country houses to paint while listening to or playing the pizzica. Other pictures took shape at popular music concerts. Her paintings are brightly coloured and depict the Salento's natural landscape, spiders and serpents, the tambourine and, frequently, a young woman [see Figs 6.1, 6.2 and 6.3). Tanya declares that she was 'bitten' in this period and became obsessed with everything that had to do with tarantism. Her tambourine, given to her as a gift by a musician, is inscribed with the words, *per Tanya, la tarantata* (for Tanya, the tarantata). In her life, she tells me, everything seemed to be going wrong. 'I'm run down,' she says. 'Does it show?'

It is 9 p.m. when we arrive at Vignacastrisi, and the town is quiet. Only the central square, bathed in yellow street lights, shows sporadic activity. The bar is open and a group of men sit on plastic chairs, chatting in the night-time shadows of a few large trees. Cars and mopeds wait by the pavement. Occasionally others drive by, cutting into the bubble of male conversations. We park next to the town hall, and a bustle of sound and movement takes us through an archway into a courtyard, where a white spotlight illuminates a rectangular space filled with some seventy chairs. A number of people intermingle and the air is filled with anticipation. The programme of the last but one of five festival days has yet to start. Tonight the Antonio Verri Award will be announced, its aim being to stimulate grass-roots creations in the fields of poetry, music and theatre.

A further hour passes. A table is set up in one corner and laid with food: bowls of freshly cut tomatoes drenched in basil and *frise*, the local dried bread. Two barrels of wine and water flank the table legs. Small groups gather, sit, talk, come and go. A cement staircase leads around two sides of the courtyard to the first floor, where two photographic exhibitions are displayed. There are pictures of the tarantate at Galatina and others of the *serpari* of San Domenico in the province of L'Aquila, Abruzzo, with processions of saintly statues and humans draped with snakes. There are also publications on sale and to give away: a collection of poems presented at previous events of this kind; short stories folded on single leaflets; and a booklet of photocopied texts and images.

By 10 p.m. a respectable crowd has assembled and a few introductory words turn one end of the courtyard into a stage. There is Annalù Sabetta, small, energetic, in a white summer dress, presenting the various performers. Tanya and her female partner are among these. In summer dresses, with painted faces, the two lay out what they identify as a magic circle. Masks, made from natural fibres, and candles mark its perimeter. Their performance evokes a mystical world, inhabited by winds and entranced beings embodied in colours, symbols, actions and songs. It is inspired, Tanya tells me later, by her recent visits to local caves. The audience, moving about freely, bridges all generations and participates keenly, looking on, chatting, commenting and applauding at the end. There are locals enjoying the evening for its out-of-the-ordinary entertainment. There are others who have come for the pizzica. Many are 'regulars' in the world of the *sibilo lungo*, the 'deep murmur', coined and identified by Antonio Verri as emanating, since time immemorial, from 'the close and profound link that exists between Salentines and their land ... that interior force which you can feel among our people, that close link with the land, which manifests itself in the grand phenomena of devotion towards our saints, our village festivals and towards the pizzica' (Presicce 1999: 11).[25] We may wonder, however, to what extent this perceived connectedness to the land and the pizzica may be generally acknowledged among Salentines or is rather a notion predominant largely among the younger and left-wing population.

The performances continue. Poetry readings alternate with short theatrical sketches and end with the declaration of the prize-winners. Tanya interrupts occasionally with theatrical gestures and elaborates on the female announcer's comments: 'Do you know Annalù? She is a tarantata like me. I ... I know her.' Remarks such as these solicit friendly amusement and feedback from the crowd. Eventually, the invited band Terra de Menzu begins to play. Only a few notes from the guitar, tambourine, flute and harmonica move the first dancers onto the floor. From the seats and side-wings others clap and sing along. Slow pieces of music alternate with faster ones. Tanya dances in the crowd and enthusiastically tries to draw others onto the floor. The fifth song is slow. The male vocalist plays with the lyrics. His gestures jokingly refer to Tanya, who is sitting next to him. The audience responds with good-hearted laughter and Tanya reacts by sensuously moving her bare shins up his leg.

The sixth piece is a pizzica. It cuts into and changes the atmosphere, propelling Tanya and others onto their feet, into its rhythm. Tanya lets out a shrill scream, throws herself onto her knees, flings her head from side to side with the tambourine's beat and imitates the tarantate's cry: 'A-hi!' Others move around and past her. She is neither ignored nor given exclusive attention as she stretches out on the ground and rolls over and over, colliding with the dancing feet of others, fingers tapping the pavement, further cries straining her vocal chords. Eventually she sits up, stands and merges with the other dancers.

The pizzica continues for over five minutes until the vocalist's sweat-covered face contorts in a grimace. He warns the other musicians and stops playing. The bleeding skin of his thumb has left blood streaks on his tambourine. Shortly afterwards the group bid farewell. Some spectators leave, too. Others remain. Chairs are moved aside to make more room. One person strikes up the chords of a song and others join in until another piece is proposed, at times interrupting the first, as musicians and audience mingle. Tanya dances, sings and plays tirelessly, communicating in grand gestures with a male singer as they improvise verses to the melody of a well-known song. By 2 a.m. the remaining participants gather around a female singer whose striking voice rings around the courtyard. At this point, Tanya and I leave. Driving home, she remarks how liberating it had been to imitate the tarantate's ritual: she feels better now.

La Sagra dei Curli presents an example of an event far from the spotlight of television cameras and media coverage. The tarantula's music and dance are engaged with to commemorate Antonio Verri and to celebrate a sense of community among his friends and fans, while endeavouring to put Verri's vision of spurring on creativity into practice, independently of predominating political tendencies or financial subsidies. It thus presents a major contrast to large-scale events in the public eye. Although unique in its objective, it may be seen as representative of many such community or home-based initiatives hosting the tarantula's music and dance, which may be recorded only in local newspapers or on home-made videos, if at all.

Clearly, just as the past ritual form of the pizzica was used not only to heal the tarantula's victims but also appropriated for manipulation and to achieve other, less explicit ends, so today the tarantula's music and dance present a double-edged sword. It is a means of advertising and merchandising the Salento – using rhetorics of musical antidotes to modern ills as a publicity scoop – without consideration of its natural and cultural heritage. At the same time, it presents not only a potential source of celebrating identities within and beyond the Salento, but also a key to developing this area according to culturally sensitive and environmentally sustainable parameters. A look at the experiences of participants, such as those of the modern tarantata Tanya reveals, moreover, how the tarantula's music and dance are still, or again, being linked to experiences of recovering well-being.

Notes

1. 'Abbasciu allu Salentu tenimu sule e mare, e cullu tamburrieddhu la gente balla e sona. Ma 'sta musica etnica ete na cartolina de nu Salentu fintu de notti e de tarante. Su etnicu 'ncazzatu percé lu tamburieddhu non deve diventare comu n anello al naso. Battitini le mani all'amministratori ca inventanu li festival e pare tutt'okei. E allora dicu ieu: mazzate pesanti culli soni e culli canti, mazzate pesanti pe' tutti senza santi. Su etnicu 'ncazzatu na cosa l'aggiu dire, se nu parlamu moi, dimme quando imu parla.'

2. Alessano, 10 August 2005. Raheli refers here to the stone walls found throughout the Salentine peninsula, made without the use of mortar from stones gathered from the rocky terrain to free land for cultivation.

3. I am not certain who first introduced this term, but it has become largely associated with the academic Piero Fumarola and some musicians, such as the group Canzoniere Grecanico Salentino, while under the direction of Daniele Durante.

4. Durante uses the term *scazzicare*.

5. In this context, Vincenzo Ampolo and Guglielmo Zappatore (1999) have also presented their research on the use of drugs in the Salento in relation to techno-pizzica experiments, as well as so-called 'counter-culture movements' and 'altered states of consciousness' more generally. Although the whiff of joints is often in the air in the context of summer pizzica concerts, some informants have stressed that the effects of drugs such as marijuana, which are likely to promote a passive attitude, are counterproductive to those of music-making or dancing, which demand active participation. More extensive research is required in this respect, but the effect of tambourines is often seen to replace and outdo even the best marijuana.

6. In 1999, there were over twenty popular music groups playing the pizzica in the Salento, of which at least five had had success elsewhere in Italy and abroad (Durante 1999: 190). By 2005, there were over fifty (Nocera 2005: 5).

7. Raf, 9 April 2004. Retrieved on 8 February 2006 from http://www. pizzicata.it/index.php?name=MDForum&file=viewtopic&t=106.

8. Lecce, 25 June 1999.

9. Piero Canizzaro's films *Ritorno a Kurumuny* (2003) and *Ritratti dal Salento* (2005) present portraits of various individuals (predominantly male) seen as *portatori* (carriers) or promoters of Salentine musical traditions.

10. This production represents the first step in a larger project signed by Cesare dell'Anna and 11/8 Records (a studio set up some years ago together with academic Piero Fumarola and musician Daniele Durante).

117

11. See 'You Tube' video clip 'Ronda di pizzica alla notte di S Rocco': http://it.youtube. com/watch?v=eJJ8gpubdTA.

12. Throughout Italy the national holiday of 15 August or ferragosto is a synonym for time off during the summer heat. Its origins go back to 18 BC when the Roman Emperor Augustus dedicated the entire month of August to festivals and celebrations (*Feriae Augusti*) and it continues to be an important Catholic holiday in honour of the Assumption of the Virgin Mary.

13. The term punkabbestia was recently included in the Italian dictionary *Nuovo Zanichelli* to indicate 'a group of young people living in the company of dogs and without a fixed home, dressing in a disorderly way and tending to have piercing and tattoos'. Often linked to the no-global and pacifist movement, this group has little in common with the transgressive 1970s London punks.

14. This campaign was launched by the Web community www.pizzicata.it.

15. For the official website, see www.lanottedellataranta.it.

16. The towns of the Grecìa Salentina include: Calimera, Carpignano Salentino, Castrignano dei Greci, Corigliano d'Otranto, Cutrofiano, Martano, Martignano, Melpignano, Soleto, Sternatia and Zollino. See http://www.greciasalentina.org/ L_Html/.

17. The following musicians have acted as musical directors of the Notte della Taranta since its inauguration: Daniele Sepe (1998); Piero Milesi (1999); Joe Zawinul (2000); Piero Milesi (2001); Vittorio Cosma (2002); Stewart Copeland (2003); Ambrogio Sparagna (2004–6); Mauro Pagani (2007–8). See Quarta (2007a).

18. The following articles are of specific relevance: Durante (1998); Fumarola (1998); Raheli (1998); Sechì (1998). See also Quarta (2007a: 18). Similar issues are developed in a series of articles published on the pizzica three years later in various editions of the *Quotidiano di Lecce* in August 2001: Blasi (2001); Di Lecce (2001a); Di Mitri (2001); Imbriani (2001); L. Santoro (2001); V. Santoro (2001).

19. See www.lanottedellataranta.it/galleria_video.php?cod=8, retrieved on 2 September 2007, for a short news report in video format on this event.

20. Lecce, 3 May 2006.

21. Lecce, 4 May 2006.

22. Two films, Piero Canizzaro's *La notte della taranta e dintorni* (2001/2003) and Paolo Pisanelli's *Il sibilo lungo della taranta* (2005), present visual documents of this event.

23. See http://aramire.splinder.com/post/9160721, retrieved 2 September 2007.

24. Verri met an untimely death in 1994 and has since acquired somewhat of a cult status among some Salentines for promoting grass-roots art and creativity.

25. 'Il sibilo lungo translates literally as "the long 's' sound", a sibilant. Although "murmur" does not capture this phoneme, it attempts to render the deep, mythic echo and murmur of the land' (Raheli 2005: 128). This notion emerges from the following much-quoted lines of Antonio Verri:
'It changes, it will change much, the face of the land, of gathered humanity, of entire towns ... what will never change is the idea of dialoguing with the earth that humanity has established from time immemorial, the long breath, 'the deep murmur' which can be heard only in the early morning, while looking out over the vast fields, while standing next to the silver trees, the silent sentinels.' (in Del Giudice 2005: 264)

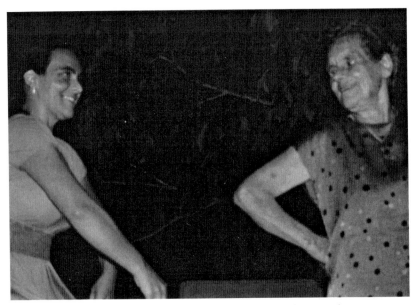

Fig. 5.1 Ada Metafune and her mother Sabina Romano dancing the pizzica, Parabita, July 2001 (photo: Karen Lüdtke).

Chapter 5
Sensing Identities and Well-being: Personal Motivations and Experiences

> To be true to oneself is, in the end, the only thread
> that links us to our individual father's house.
> It's our true identity: idem, the same, that which remains,
> even when the circumstances change.

> Eugenio Barba, Lecce, 11 November 2002[1]

'The success of the pizzica today is directly linked to the fact that tarantism no longer exists,' says one middle-aged Salentine man, suggesting that show business grows on the negation of crises and cure.[2] One exits and the other enters on stage, and their appearances appear irreconcilable. Would tarantism, with its heavy baggage of inherent crises and suffering, make it to the headlines today if it were too close to the bone, if it were attributed more than a soap opera feel? The answer of a middle-aged woman, native to Galatina is clear: 'Today this tradition has lost itself. It was more than a tradition; it was anguish. We experienced it above all as anguish. But today you don't feel that any more. I find it interesting as something that identifies us as Salentines. But I wouldn't take up anything other than the dance for today's purposes.'[3] Nowadays, it appears most people in the Salento would defend this view. According to its new terms and new outfit as a source of local pride and identity, tarantism can resurface even within officially religious and political contexts.

Very few speak openly about the crises cutting into their lives today and how they relate these to their engagement with the pizzica and other Salentine music. Every performance is, however, cross-cut by the personal biography of each participant, and every stage, no matter how publicized or intimate, is set within a complex web of intentions and choices. The current media hype leaves little, if any, space or attention for the personal dimensions behind this buzz, some explicit, others tucked away in the wings. A number of Salentines, however, like Tanya, who danced at the Sagra dei Curli in 1998, link their experiences of the pizzica to sensations of enhanced well-being. A consideration of the individual motivations and experiences of performers engaging in the tarantula's music and dance today reveals how memories, autobiographies and perceptions of the self may be evoked, reshaped and reconstituted in this way.

The group Alla Bua, perhaps more than any other, has linked its performances to discourses on well-being. Their focus on the healing power of the tarantula's music, although emphasized less in recent years, sets the scene for the accounts of two women, Tanya Pagliara and Ada Metafune, whose lives have been transformed through their engagement with the tarantula.

The Alla Bua: Music for Healing

On 24 April 1998, I see the Alla Bua on stage, in action. On this occasion, what at first seems a technical disaster brings home to me aspects of what these musicians define as the potential of their music. It is Friday evening; the group is up on an elevated stage in a large tent-like sports hall in the town of Taurisano in the south-west Salento. The floor before them is packed with teenagers dancing to their fast and frenzied rhythms. Then, suddenly, the electric fuses blow and, as the amplifiers go out, the music jumps to a different volume and tonality, ringing, for a moment, through the dark, until dim emergency lights reset the scene. The atmosphere has changed and the musicians have moved forward from behind their now-useless, microphones. They step off the stage without interrupting their playing and begin to circle the dance floor. Then they halt in a semicircle and suddenly turn round.

All at once, a young female participant finds herself trapped in a ring of pounding instruments. She remains frozen, standing as she had before, with her arms folded protectively across her chest. The musicians play fiercely, letting their instruments address her, their eyes making no contact with hers. She laughs back, embarrassed, at others joking about the trap she is in. A moment later, one of her legs starts to move to the beats that are bombarding her, and her arms slip open, dropping to her side. After no more than a minute or two the musicians turn away and move on around the dance space. Freed from their clasp, the young woman joins the crowd of dancers. Later she tells me:

> I had been feeling angry, after an argument with a friend, and was standing on my own, trapped in my anger and closed stance. The musicians took me by surprise. Their music provoked an itch to dance, to get rid of the iron grip of this contained rage excluding me from dancing. By standing round me, physically cutting me off from the dance floor, this sense of confinement was duplicated, externalized. At the same time, the music encouraged a reaction and, like an invitation, drew me out of my frozen state. In fact, as soon as the musicians moved away, I joined in the dancing without a second thought, my anger pushed backstage by the desire to dance, to be part of the fun.

When I relate this occasion to the lead singer and tambourine player of the group Alla Bua, at a later date, he replies:

> Our music has a certain force. It is a force. A successful performance starts off slowly and then gradually we try to charge the music more and more, always more, increasing the rhythm. A strong sense of flying is evoked. Sometimes it rises up directly from the feet. You feel the music physically. When I feel this sensation, in that moment, I'm happy, I'm content. It is something that gives me immense pleasure, because I know then that if I am feeling these vibrations, these sensations, the others are feeling them too. However, when I don't feel this sensation – this music that takes off by itself – I feel discontented, I feel down. But, to us, it almost always happens! Even though we aren't musicians. I don't know music. I've studied it by myself, but I don't know how to play an instrument. I know how to play the tambourine, but it doesn't have particular chords, ours at least. It's not based on notes, but on tonality and vibrations. To trust in your own force, potency and spirituality means succumbing with this force and spirituality to everything that you don't know on a theoretical and practical level as far as music is concerned.[4]

The three group members I spoke to were all in their mid to late forties at the time.[5] Two of them grew up with the pizzica. Playing this music, they argue, has always been an important part of their lives and their identity. The third is a psychologist who is originally from the Salento but spent many years of his childhood and student life in other parts of Italy before settling back in the Salento.

123

Inevitably, the outlook and aim of this group has been influenced by his various insights into the curative uses of music in other cultural and therapeutic contexts.

'Their way of understanding and playing music aims to involve the spectator in a frenetic and liberating dance which helps to cure "modern ills": stress, tension, anxiety, depression, etc.' (Anon. 2002). Such is the presentation of the Alla Bua in a summer events calendar. Assumptions linking the pizzica and well-being merge with others expressed in the group's first 2003 music video (Alla Bua 2003): this portrays ritual re-enactments of transparently dressed teenage tarantate responding, with pouting lips and swaying hips, to the insistent drumming and piercing gaze of male musicians. Highly charged erotic images speak for themselves, showing how modern life reverberates both to the beat of industrial and commercial demands and to images of femininity and masculinity as portrayed in fashion magazines and TV spots. Nevertheless, concert settings are – often uncritically – attributed a healing potential, and the pizzica is seen to maintain therapeutic powers capable of addressing contemporary afflictions.

'They say that we play "hard pizzica"!' affirms the Alla Bua lead singer. 'It's because of the intense and fast manner in which we play'.[6] 'The rhythms today are different,' the group's guitarist explains further:

That is why we express this music differently. They tell us that we play 'pizzica rock'. Why? Because this attracts the young people. Clearly, it is also a personal form of expression, our way of interpreting the pizzica. But, at the same time, we've noticed that this form is closer to the music of teenagers today, who also live in more accelerated terms. In my opinion, it is this that makes this music a form of therapy, because it links the ancient – our musical tradition, which entails certain values – with faster rhythms, which are those of today. It reunites our traditions and origins with how we live today. It gives the young teenagers a sense of continuity, while they live in a schizophrenic manner, with extreme generational and cultural gaps. They immediately throw themselves into these frenetic rhythms, not knowing what their origins are. But musically and rhythmically they live these rhythms as resonances inside themselves, whether in a conscious or unconscious manner.[7]

All three musicians confirm that they see a link between the music they are playing and its impact on well-being. One of them expands on this:

> Yes, because it does us good as well. For us, too, the same method as for the tarantate can be used. It's the same. Music is important because it's like an outstretched hand. The rhythm is like a hand that helps you get up when you don't feel well, when you're ill, when you can't walk properly; it repairs you. Music summons up energy, it calls upon the spirit or, rather, I'd use the word blood; it calls upon the blood, just like a magnet. This is the message we try to communicate. It's very simple. We invite everyone to communicate, because we feel the need for this energy to circulate, to be able to feel it within our spirits, in order to feel well.[8]

This link between music and well-being is also seen to be expressed in the group's name:

> The name Alla Bua may be seen to mean 'other cure'. The name may have many meanings. We called ourselves the Alla Bua initially because we often played in a tavern, where a group of old men, when singing, always repeated these words as a refrain between the verses of whatever song they were singing. It never came to my mind to ask them why. However, first of all, what is the meaning of *la bua*? It means fracture, confusion, and abrasion, something that has hurt you. Meanwhile, our music can have a therapeutic effect. There is therefore this sense of fracture, and at the same time the notion of healing.[9]

Like the Alla Bua musicians, two modern tarantate describe the impacts of the tarantula's music and dance, as promoting well-being.

Tanya's Story: Dancing Colours

I first met Tanya, who re-enacted elements of the tarantate's rituals at the Sagra dei Curli in August 1998, when she was in her early thirties. At the time, she was studying to complete her university degree in sociology and actively following her vocation as a painter, while living with her mother in a village just outside Lecce. Her life story is marked by disjunctures: her parents were separated and she spent various periods of residence between Italy and France, where her father lived. When I meet Tanya again in February 2008, she confirms that her need for the tarantula's music and dance, animating the creation of her paintings [see Figs 6.1, 6.2 and 6.3], was directly linked to a love story that could not be expressed or lived due to the circumstances within which it emerged. She associates this with the time of her initial bite. On 27 January 1998, during a visit to her home near Lecce, Tanya first told me the following:

> We were painting in the open, on the beach, with music at a high volume. It was a type of techno situation. There were lots of young people, playing the *djembe* and tambourines. There was absolute liberty. The heat was terrible. I was barefoot all day long. We were living in direct contact with nature, always hearing those primordial, archaic rhythms, dum, dum, dum. And I felt this bite, the bite of this earth. At the time, I accessed a magic world of my own.
>
> In retrospect, a year on, I have tried to rationalize it all. I think that something was moved inside me, repressed memories, all of the culture I received when young, the fear of the tarantula. Seeing and visualizing this phobia in something else, in an artistic product, unchained this reaction in me. But also a love story, because guilt followed, remorse, the figure of the Salentine woman with everything she entails. There was this fear of being bitten by a spider since I was small, then the fact of not believing in anything when I was older, and then the experience of entering into this absurd dimension. I believed in the tarantula. I felt possessed, but possessed in a strange way, because there was a lucid part of me that didn't believe in anything.
>
> It all began two years ago when I decided to follow a university course in the sociology of religions.[10] I went sporadically and with little interest. However, hearing and speaking about tarantism, about altered states of consciousness, about Castaneda, and seeing videos about these topics, inspired me to find out whether there was someone who was expressing these things artistically: a tarantolated painter ... I met him, a painter from Gallipoli, who feels the bite of this earth. He has read a lot of Castaneda and, in an artistic manner, expresses the feel of this land and the bite of the Salentine earth. His favourite subjects are tarantulas or crabs, things that bite. He says that he speaks with the snakes and has always felt this call, this strange bite.
>
> I suspected that it had to do with phenomena of trances linked to images: seeing the painting of the other artist, I entered into this dimension. He maintains that the inducing factor was the loud music played all day long under the burning sun and the hard work that made us access these images, this other dimension of consciousness. There are many factors. I can't tell you what it was exactly. I followed the tambourine players, all of the groups. For an entire year, I did performances with them. I wasn't in a lucid state, although there was a lucid part of me which knew that I had to follow that road, to get out of this, to become rational again,

because I was living only off colours and sounds. All day long I was fixed on hearing the tambourines. I passed from psychedelic art to this typically Salentine thing, even though I don't feel Salentine. I have lived here, in France, in Sardinia. Maybe it was the influence the university course had on me regarding tarantism and altered states of consciousness. I associated these with the type of painting I was doing before, the psychedelic art of the discos. Previously, I had never painted typically Salentine subjects. This must have been the input.

I told myself, you can do it, but only by tarantulating yourself, as a tarantolata. I'm not sure if I liked it or not, because many of those things happened to me which you cannot talk about, which cannot be said in words. I became part of a magic game. I decided to leave, to go to Paris, to stay there for three months to try and liberate myself, and when I returned I decided to create *l'arcu pintu*,[11] to work in a group, as therapy, to get out of this dimension. I looked for other artists who had something of me. We went into the countryside, to abandoned farmhouses. We didn't eat. We listened only to the tambourines. There was a strange contact between the seven members of our group. We didn't communicate. We understood each other in our own way and we created our pictures in this primordial state.

Before continuing, Tanya takes me to a back room where she has stored her paintings. There are over twenty animated by a spider in some part or other of the frame. The colours are bright, oils mixed with earth and other natural fibres, and some of the canvases stretch up to a metre or two in length and breath. One by one, Tanya holds up her pictures and speaks about what inspired her to create each one:

This picture shows an olive tree that is spitting out a tambourine. It is the sensation of the tarantula: an ugly olive tree that is vomiting a tambourine, a vortex that turns and turns. I made this while I was in a trance. There's lots of movement. It's rhythmical. They told me that I was dancing while painting. But the idea didn't come to me. My consciousness was completely annihilated. I was concentrating on those sounds of the tambourines. I didn't feel anything. I opened my eyes and saw this image. It had materialized itself. I didn't conceive it beforehand. It exploded in my head on its own and I discharged it, onto the earth.

And I got out of that dimension. It was a real therapy in the end to collaborate with the others. I gave a part of myself. I encouraged the others to live in the way that I was living. I entered into a dimension of myself and the others. I – us – God. That is not I – God. But, we – God. We – God – I. Among all artists there is this predominance of thinking: 'I against the others' or 'I am my own God.' Instead, being together we created an 'I-

127

individual-but-group'. We tried to understand what was meant by this *ballo all'arcu pintu*, this dance of the arcu pintu, which is often referred to with respect to the tarantate. That is, to dance a colour, what does it mean? This is what we experienced in the end. We felt the arcu pintu inside ourselves, as a visualization. It's something that cannot be said in words. You feel, see and touch the sounds and colours. It is a different dimension of awareness, where sound and colours become mixed and quasi-materialized.[12]

Later, when I recovered, I enquired about the meaning of the term arcu pintu. I wanted to understand what these colours of tarantism were. Why did the women see all the colours, wanting to dance all the colours, all the emotions? What I was told, although these things are never certain, is that arcu pintu is derived from the *arcu dellu pintu*, which refers to weaving in colours, like the spider. A woman weaves her cloth with specific colours, with specific emotions, maybe the particular emotion that has made her ill. For some, arcu pintu implied something mystic linked to Salentine magic, something that the spirits have, to hide treasures, mischievous spirits who play with destiny; for others, this term referred to architecture, to a painted arch; for yet others, it implied the rainbow, seven frequencies, seven colours. This is what the old people told me. For the young people it doesn't mean anything. For me it relates everything, like a keyword.

From the moment that you enter into this world of the tarantate, etc., you find yourself thinking as a believer, as a Catholic, as a superstitious person. Then you think, no, it's not possible. There is something strange, time flows differently, the circle always repeats itself, an absurd circle repeats itself, strange encounters, for instance, or knowing in advance where a person is, meeting a number of people all interested in the same things at a single site. It's something that can't be said in words. For a believer it is a saint, destiny, the tarantula. I believe that it is strong suggestion, which induces this dimension where space and time change and consequently you live in another way. The contact between people, space, time and the others changes, and then these quasi-mystical things happen. It is mysticism, even though mysticism is different. Others also see me as someone mystical, magical, but I don't feel that way. Every time somebody experiences modified states of consciousness, they begin to speak in mystical terms. For that reason I've also been taken for a kind of saint. It annoys me, because it's not like that.

Tanya struggles to describe what she has lived. Her account underlines the difficulty of conveying subjective experiences in words. Metaphors and symbols help, but their multivalency inevitably invites diverging interpretations and misunderstandings. Like Ada and Matteo on 29 June 2001 in Galatina and the tarantate in the past, Tanya weaves meaningful links between apparent coincidences. She draws, moreover, not only on the phenomenon of tarantism, but also on anthropological, sociological and New Age literature, grasping the notions of magic, mysticism, trance and altered states of consciousness in an attempt to express what she has experienced. She goes on:

> In our group, l'arcu pintu, we spoke a lot about our experiences, about altered states of consciousness and about whether art was therapy for us or not. What emerged is that it is a form of therapy, yes, but not alone. There is this desire to recompose our sense of self, which is torn from the existing social system, because no artist recognizes herself in this social system. However, art goes beyond therapy: it is a message, a way of communicating with others and for some it is a way of communicating with God, for others a means of contesting, of upsetting the existing culture, of creating a counter-culture with images. In this sense, it goes beyond therapy, but there is also therapy. Therapy is above all socialization, an alternative way of socializing for artists. We socialized in this way. That was the beautiful thing about l'arcu pintu: we came out of our shells, our worlds, our individualism that is typical of painters. Instead, l'arcu pintu as a group was an alternative group, an alternative way of socializing. There was therapy, because I didn't manage to get out of this state on my own. I wanted to return to normality to communicate with others. In this sense there was therapy, not because I wasn't well in this situation, but because I couldn't survive in it.
>
> The alternative would have been to become an artist on the street, that's all. I knew Edoardo, who had chosen this life of a completely liberated artist, of a savage.[13] It was he who made me understand that, if I continued on this road, I would never become anything. A bohemian artist today would serve no purpose. In fact, he advised me to alternatively enter and leave the social order, to live altered states of consciousness, but also to then find a way of entering the social system again and of creating a role for myself, even if it was a feigned one; not only one role, but several roles, to be able to completely annihilate consciousness, to pursue only my instinct and to express myself only with colours, but then also to be capable of assuming a well-defined role and entering the system. In this sense, l'arcu pintu was therapy, a way of returning to everyday consciousness.[14]

Tanya refers to recovering a greater sense of well-being through forms of socialization and through experiences of reality seen to be different from those of everyday life. She speaks of a sense of fragmentation, an experience of being torn from the system, which she sees as characterizing the existence of artists like herself. The process of re-integration into society is what she identifies as recovery: not because she wasn't well before, in the period she described herself as 'bitten', but because she realized that in today's society she couldn't survive in this way. In this sense recovery required a compromise. It involved finding others with whom she could share an experience of well-being, suspending and eliminating her feelings of being disjointed. It also involved a shift in perspective: Tanya speaks of the need to play roles in order to belong in and fit into the existing social order, even if she may not always condone it. Her self-reflexive attempts to rationalize her experiences linked to the tarantula have made her increasingly conscious of the flexibility of the roles she plays and of their ability to rewrite and transform her sense of self.

When we meet again in 2008, Tanya is still painting, as well as writing about her own experiences in relation to the tarantula. Although the spider may have lost some of its pertinence in her life, it continues to serve as a channel of expression. Meanwhile, Ada's story too is one of recovery, of retrieving a sense of empowerment and a growing awareness of an identity beyond affliction.

Ada's Story: Retrieving Soundness

Three days after performing the tarantula's dance for the cameras of Canale 5 on 29 June 2001, the very day she had gone to Galatina and witnessed Matteo and Evelina's displays of crises, Ada tells me how she had lived this experience:

> Afterwards, I felt very empty. In the past, I tried to do something to make this go away. I became afraid. Now I confront it with more calmness. That's the way it is. I let the emptiness be. I didn't do anything to send it away. I listened to it with some sadness. You give a large part of yourself. It's the same sensation as when you give a very strong workshop. It's similar. The days afterwards I felt overwhelmed. I have physical bruises because it was very hard on the ground and I hurt myself a little. Today it is different from fifty years ago. The tarantate of the past did it without awareness. They knew they would be better. For someone who knows, the impact is even stronger. This time it was different from the other times. I knew I was going towards something and I knew I would confront it with awareness. In tarantism a degree of awareness always remains, even if it seems to you that you do not have any dimension of body or soul. For those of us who have lived closure – let's say for me, because I can speak only for myself – it has a profound significance.[15]

Ada speaks of being overwhelmed by a sense of emptiness and closure, as in some way juxtaposed – or complementary? – to the experience of herself as without limits, without body or soul, while re-enacting the tarantate's ritual. The clarity and calm with which she now speaks have emerged from her story marked by periods of crises. She had first told me about these two years earlier:

> I started to dance in my early twenties on the occasions when the pizzica was played. My father was against it. It was not seen as a very respectable thing to do. But I felt the need to dance on every occasion that presented itself. Just like the tarantate in the past. Looking back, I now see how this process of learning to dance changed me. My childhood led me to rationalize everything. My emotions and my body were practically non-existent for me. However, when I began to dance, everything around me disappeared and I instinctively began to communicate with my body. At festivals and concerts, others began to acknowledge me as someone who dances well. I was invited to work with a performance group. On stage, I had to learn to open myself to the audience. Before I had always felt embarrassed about my body. I wanted to be taller and slimmer. I had tried to hide my breasts. The birth of my first child left me completely disintegrated. I did psychoanalysis for a while and stopped again. But, I continued to dance. I'd forget about everything around. It was a way of presenting myself as I was. It helped me to gain security about my body and to express my feelings.
>
> With the pizzica pizzica, you can live out all of your sensuality. It is you who direct the dance, subtly, even though it is the man who circles around you. Learning the scherma was a final step for me. It is all about defining and defending your territory. It forced me to bring out the aggression which I'd always hidden before. Through dancing, I not only regained access to my emotions but also to an energy which we have inside and which is part of something larger, something global. I don't think that such a force, brought alive when you dance, can be accidental. There must be an underlying layer that nourishes it. Although for a long time I avoided the Church, I now believe in a spirituality that is universal, that doesn't classify faiths.[16]

Dancing on public occasions and to live music allowed Ada to come to acknowledge her own body and her emotions, as she says [see Fig. 5.1]. While her father and elderly villagers had discouraged her from dancing and communicating in this way, she experienced others admiring and appreciating her talent at concerts of the tarantula's music and dance. Moreover, experiences of dancing were influential in transforming her initial resistance towards the Catholic

Church into an openness towards a sacred dimension, which she now sees as inherent in nature and reality at large.

In 2001, Ada spoke to me again about the pizzica in her life:

> You know, it's simply that it doesn't end here. Now I'm more aware of what happens but I still always have to try not to live in a split state. It's a continuous journey. And I have little time to myself. For me, today, emptiness is really the key. Even today I often find myself rationalizing everything, to cut myself off from the head downwards. And it's not always easy to reunite that which I am. Even today I often ask myself: who am I?
>
> Everything started a bit with my marriage. I was twenty-nine. It was perfect. But I didn't feel anything. Nothing. For two years afterwards, I kept myself under control. Then some psychosomatic symptoms started. My head was spinning. I felt unwell. But the doctors didn't find physical reasons to explain my affliction.[17] Then, when my son was born, everything exploded. Until that point, I had everything under control. But it was as if everything was already going towards this culmination.
>
> Today, ten years later, I am calmer. With the family, I don't have much time for myself. But the children also help me, because they are very spontaneous. With their reactions they make me reflect about myself. At the beginning I wanted to throw away everything that I'd been, that had been a part of my life. I had to accept parts of myself that I didn't like and I got to know other aspects that I didn't know before.[18]

As Ada speaks her young son becomes increasingly agitated. He asks his mother to help him put in a video and to stop talking so he can follow the sound of the film. 'He doesn't like me to talk about these things,' Ada explains. 'He immediately gets angry.' No doubt it raised red flags of difficult times. Five years later, in April 2006, when I ask Ada whether she would prefer me to use a pseudonym to tell her story, her answer is very clear: 'No, this is who I am.'

Clearly, the accounts of Tanya, Ada and the Alla Bua provide snapshots of intricate biographies, which need to be considered in relation to the lives of others who may or may not see themselves as modern tarantati, in order to examine what patterns may be identified among pizzica enthusiasts more generally. Ada's story, meanwhile, like Tanya's, raises questions about whether she would have experienced the impact of the pizzica as powerfully as she relates had it not been paralleled with the boom of the tarantula's music and dance. How effective, moreover, can the appropriation of the tarantula's symbolism be considering its inherent historical fracture? Even if Tanya found a sense of belonging within her group of artist friends, did this permeate her life more generally? Even if Ada has gained recognition as a dancer both on and off stage – and as one of the few female scherma dancers, if not the only one, performing at Torrepaduli – to what extent has this reconciled her with wider society, within which tarantism has become a free-for-all gadget? And to what degree is the therapeutic rhetoric of the Alla Bua accepted and defended by others – whether musicians or not?

Although the experiences and views described here may apply only to a minority of those engaging with the tarantula's music and dance today, what transpires is that, while the 1990s boom of the pizzica may be directly linked to the death of tarantism in its traditional sense, it has nevertheless been re-appropriated by some contemporary performers to promote discourses and experiences of well-being. Just as the tarantate's crises referred to highly varied personal circumstances linked to the inability to cope, so the stories of Tanya and Ada relate diverse experiences of crises, leaving both women incapable of coping with their lives on the basis of the explanatory frameworks available to them. By engaging with the pizzica in their own idiosyncratic ways, but within a context in which this music and dance were gaining popularity on a daily basis, the two women found relief. Ada speaks of coping with emptiness now. Tanya tells of coming to terms with ways of socializing in daily life. These personal accounts demand a look at how meanings, explanatory systems and treatment options were and are negotiated, on a more general level, to identify those under the tarantula's spell.

Notes

1. University of Lecce. This is a citation from a talk given by Eugenio Barba, founder of the International School of Theatre Anthropology, during a workshop entitled '*La casa di mio padre*' (My Father's House), stressing Barba's Salentine origins.

2 Lecce, 14 October 2005.

3 Galatina, 24 June 1999.

4. 29 May 1998.

5. Two of its members have left the group Alla Bua since the time of these interviews.

6. 29 May 1998.

7. 7 May 1998.

8. 20 May 1998.

9. 29 May 1998. For an explanation of the group's name, see also www.allabua.it: 'The meaning, it would seem, comes from the ancient Greek language (truly ancient, from the Lower Salento, and not the area called Grecìa today, circumscribed by some ten municipalities and quite far from Alliste, the place of this discovery): Alla Bua stands for alternative medicine, other cure.' Retrieved on 30 September 2007 from http://www.allabua.it/09_gruppo.html.

10 A similar example of the role of academics and university seminars in the tarantula's contemporary web, both as a source of information and initial instigator – or metaphorical 'first bite' – is given by Maurizio Nocera's interview with Tore Greco. When asked about the occasion on which he first felt the spider's presence, Tore responds: 'There is a precise point of reference: the presence of Georges Lapassade in Lecce on the occasion of the seminar 'Il ragno del dio che danza' (the spider of the god who dances) at the Salentine university' (Nocera 2005: 45).

11. This term literally means 'painted arch' and was the name Tanya gave to the group of artists referred to here.

12. Tanya mentions a phenomenon commonly associated with experiences of so-called altered states of consciousness in which cross-sensory impulses are triggered: 'a colour can be heard, a sound can be seen' (Lapassade 1996a: 169). This neurologically based phenomenon, also known as synaesthesia or synethesia, literally meaning 'joining the senses', implies that one type of sensory stimulation elicits the automatic, involuntary stimulation of another.

13. Tanya refers to the late Salentine artist Edoardo De Candia, known for his unconventional lifestyle and choice to partly live in nudity (Massari 1998).

14. 27 January 1998.

15. 2 July 2001.

16. 19 August 1999. The account presented here is a summary of Ada's responses to my question about the impact of dancing on her life.
17. Ada, just like the tarantato Francesco Greco, uses the term *il mio male* to refer to her crises.
18. 25 July 2001.

Part III
From Ritual to Limelight

Moving on to a comparison of the tarantula's music and dance in historical and contemporary contexts reveals underlying factors influencing self-perceptions, human relations, power issues and visions of reality sabotaging or nourishing well-being. Chapter 6, 'Spider WoMen Transfixed', explores what labels and world views defined and diagnosed the tarantate and what criteria can be seen to characterize their contemporary namesakes. This shows how, in the modern Salento, the tarantula's music and dance leave their imprint on forms of deeper-lying suffering existing under new headings today. Chapter 7, 'Tarantula Threads and Showbiz Airs,' is a tightrope walk between past and present performative places, times, props and techniques, balancing out what were and are subtle clues to performative success. The right music, in the sense of appropriate and efficacious, had and has to be found. The aim was and is to facilitate participation. The props were and are communal and entail the potential side effects of manipulation and exploitation. Yet key differences stand out, as Chapter 8, 'SpiderWoMen Transformed,' reveals. In the past tarantism rituals allowed for the expression of extreme emotional crises. Although this is rarely the case today, the tarantula's music and dance may affect participants' daily lives, fostering a sense of 'magic', rhythmic synchrony, sensuality and well-being through exposure to new experiences and insights, perceived to beneficially influence perceptions of the self, others and the world at large.

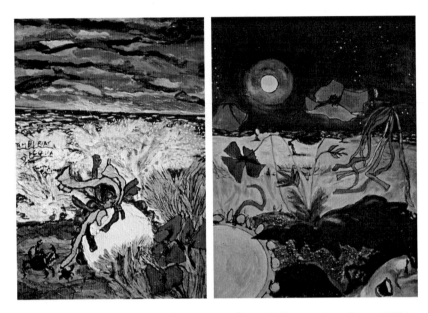

Figs 6.1, 6.2 and 6.3 Paintings by Tanya Pagliara, Collezione Arcu Pintu, 1997 (6.3 © Tanya Pagliara. Reproduced with permission of Daniele Durante).

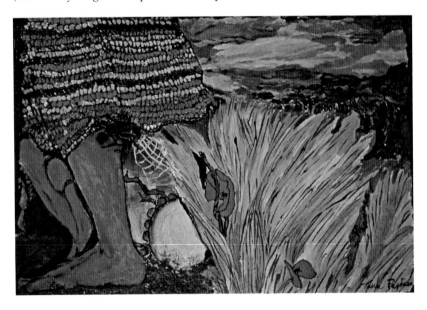

Chapter 6
Spider WoMen Transfixed: Negotiating Crisis and Cure

> The NEO-TARANTATA ... could be concealed inside your sister, cousin, supermarket assistant, dentist's secretary or university colleague. As a remedy to quotidian life, they have decided that there is nothing better than to toss themselves about in the centre of a circle of tambourines or in front of a hi-fi system in public to help them remove the stress of everyday life. We are dealing with girls ... from good families, without any psychological problem or social drama behind them other than the tragedy of having too much free time on their hands.
>
> Francesco Patruno (2003)

With his conspicuous sense of humour, Patruno (2003) takes a provocative stance, stressing that the focus on recovering well-being through the tarantula's music and dance brought into relief in this study is highly ambiguous. This view questions whether and to what extent we may compare those transfixed by the tarantula spider in past and present times.

In this context, anthropological studies on health and illness have increasingly challenged the contours and assumptions of biomedicine, revealing that 'non-medical healing is empirical in the sense that it is often based on systematic observation and interpretation of symptoms, suffering, cause, effects and response to treatment' (Csordas and Kleinman 1996: 5). The tarantula's ritual too was grounded in experiential knowledge, transmitted, tested, re-evaluated and adapted over many generations.

Acknowledgement of such experience-based knowledge relies heavily on a recognition of the body as both objectively and subjectively – and therefore also socially and politically – founded. Increasingly, anthropological work on the body and embodiment has revealed the phenomenological, social and political dimensions of the human organism (Scheper-Hughes and Lock 1987), and underlined the need to consider bio-medicine as one culturally specific system of cure, whose basic precepts are fundamentally challenged by anthropological stances: 'Whereas biomedicine, in theory if not always in practice, presupposes a universal, a historical subject, critically interpretative medical anthropologists are confronted with rebellious and "anarchic" bodies – bodies that refuse to conform (or submit) to presumably universal categories and concepts of diseases, distress and medical efficacy' (Lock and Scheper-Hughes 1996: 41–43). As the human organism is engaged on a phenomenological, social and political level, an analysis of healing practices, such as the tarantula's cult, must include a consideration of the negotiative process that takes place between these various dimensions. How does this process weave threads of meaning and relations that re-anchor the individual in their own body, as well as in the social and natural worlds?

Answers begin to emerge if we explore, first, how individuals came and come to be characterized as someone who was 'bitten by the tarantula'; secondly, what world views and perceptions of affliction and well-being underlie such a definition or diagnosis; and, finally, how treatment options concern choices that were and are available and – just as important – acceptable.

Diagnosing Spiders: Identifying Tarantula Cases

First, I look into the eyes and, if it's there, the poison can be seen. Secondly, vibrations show whether a person is stirred up or not. Thirdly, you look at the tips of the toes, because the toes don't remain still. You feel a sense of electrification, different from a nervous attack, which is temporary. If I don't notice these things, it is pointless to go and play.

In this way, Luigi Stifani, musician of the tarantate, identified those under the tarantula's spell (Chiriatti 1995: 49).

In the past, moments of affliction varied: on rare occasions, a physical bite was actually registered. Alternatively, a spider, or other venomous creature, was encountered, in waking life or in a dream. At times, it was enough to be brushed by the breath, *il soffio*, of a snake. Moreover, someone may have been 'infected' by the contagious influence of others. The physical rhythms of trembling, shaking and convulsions of one tarantata appeared to create a vibrational impact on others. In the absence of a clear cause, meanwhile, cases were identified in a process of auto-diagnosis or with the help of those familiar with the symptoms involved.

Without doubt, these criteria depend on experiential know-how. De Martino (2005: 58) adds the intolerance of some tarantate to certain dishes or smells, frequent dreams of serpents or of St Paul, and an overall heightened sensitivity to music. Moreover, popular opinion characterized the tarantula's victims as possessed by an 'irresistible urge to dance', as musical and chromatic explorations established the tarantula's involvement. Clearly, an identification of symptoms required a basic agreement between the afflicted and others about what kind of problem was at hand and what kind of treatment was deemed appropriate.

Language gives another avenue of access to how the tarantate perceived and described themselves. While the term tarantism belongs to the jargon of scholars, Salentine people speak of someone who holds the tarantula (*tiene la taranta*), was stung (*è stata pizzicata*) or is a tarantata (*è una tarantata*). They are those, De Martino (2005: 37–38) tells, whom the tarantula *fa scazzicare*, excites or arouses. Uncontrollable erotic impulses are often referred to in this way. 'This summer I will become a tarantula!' a young Salentine musician told me fervently in June 1999, expressing his frustration about never having had a sexual encounter with a woman.[1] I ask what he means by this. He explains: 'Qualcosa che mi scazzica!' (Something that excites me!) Evelina's grandson uses the same word to describe his grandmother when taken over by crises: 'Si scazzica!'[2] '*Scazzicare* also denotes a difficulty in standing up (*mi scàzzicu*, I stand up with difficulty)', De Martino (2005: 38) specifies, and 'appears to symbolize the state of inertia, prostration and weariness which, together with a disorderly motor release, makes up the "crisis" moment of tarantism'. Feeling bored (*annoiato*), injured (*leso*), fractured (*spezzato*) or broken (*rotto*) were other ways the tarantate described their afflictions (De Martino 2005: 56–57, 91).

One informant talked of her tarantulated grandmother as consistently tense, bearing a weight on her shoulders.[3] Yet others speak of a state of tedium or boredom, *un stato di noia*. One tarantata reported spiders crawling underneath her pillow at night.[4] Another talked of feeling ants in different parts of the body,[5] while a male tarantato claimed that there was a spider in his right testicle. In May and June, the sensation of having a swarm or ants' nest, *un formicolio* ('pins and needles'), inside this testicle was at its worst, preventing him from having an orgasm. However, eventually the spider travelled down the leg, remaining in the right big toe until its resurgence the following year (Nocera 2005: 45–64). Most tarantate, Maurizio Nocera argues, moreover, do not see their bodies as something pleasing.[6]

Anthropological work has widely considered how humans perceive animals in relation to how they experience their bodies or themselves (Douglas 1966; Sperber 1996). Spiders, like insects, are generally seen to fall into ambiguous or anomalous categories, defying any clear distinctions. Although much confusion exists about exactly what spider was the culprit in the case of tarantism, perceptions of the tormenting tarantula, Ioan Lewis (1991: 516–17) argues, draw from the zoological characteristics of two types of spiders that were, and to a minor degree still are, part of the Salentine fauna: *Lycosa tarantula* and *Latrodectus tredecim guttatus*. *Latrodectus*, more commonly known as Malmignatte or European black widow, is a small spider, which awaits its prey in its web.[7] The female's bite causes severe, although rarely lethal, general reactions afflicting the entire body and these are the symptoms on which the acute crises of the tarantate appear to be modelled. Meanwhile, the visually impressive *Lycosa tarantula* is a large, black, hairy spider, which lives underground and is equipped with threatening claws to hunt its prey. It stands, according to Lewis, as a key contestant for the spirit spider believed to be responsible for the tarantate's affliction, on the basis of its appearance and the striking local symptoms of its bite. Although its poison causes no discernible general effects, the *Lycosa*'s bite leaves a large, red, swollen mark on the skin surface. The mythic spider thus incorporates, as social anthropologist David Parkin observes, a dual ambivalence derived from the small but spiteful *Latrodectus* and the large, aggressive but harmless *Lycosa*.[8]

Spiders and their poisons penetrate and jeopardize bodily boundaries, threatening the safety net of perceived stability. 'They appear as the symbols of creative formlessness, of loss of control; they have the power to overturn the established order' (Berman 1990: 81–82), bringing to the surface further analogies: the liminal status of the spider may be a metaphor for the liminal experience of illness (poised between health and death) itself. Views of illness as externally caused, moreover, create phenomenological associations between subjective experience and broader social and cultural landscapes, making family and community members – as significant actors in this broader play – intrinsic to the healing process. Music, meanwhile, equally liminal – in the sense of ephemeral – and capable of penetrating the body, embodies the potential for recovery.[9]

But what about today? Can we speak of a diagnosis, in the sense of identifying criteria characterizing the modern tarantati? Various terms are used in the Salento today (at times seriously, at times jokingly) to forge a link between today's pizzica fans and the tarantate of yesteryear. People speak of the neo-tarantati, nuovi tarantati, modern tarantati or *attarantati*. Some distinguish today's tarantati from the tarantolati of the past, but these definitions are by no means unanimous. Often meanings are conflated, without much thought for underlying epistemological implications. 'I don't know how to define myself,' music teacher, dancer and self-acclaimed tarantata Maria Antonietta Epifani (1998) wonders. 'Perhaps it's simply the need to dance; the inability to remain still when I hear a tambourine play.'[10] 'I always dance', one skilled singer and dancer adds, 'with all kinds of music: the pizzica, Arabic music, African music. I'm a tarantata: an international tarantata!'[11] Such an 'urge to dance' may inevitably refer to a spectrum of motives and meanings. According to this criterion, most young children are contemporary tarantati as they are generally the first, least inhibited and most persistent dancers at pizzica concerts. In fact, the group Canzoniere Grecanico Salentino dedicated one of its lullabies – with lyrics evoking the tarantula – to 'all the children of the Salento, who are tarantati like ourselves'.[12]

Others subtly differentiate possible affinities with the tarantate of the past.[13] Daniele Durante writes: 'The new "tarantati" are not possessed by anything or anyone, but nevertheless are in search of a god (or demon?)' (1999: 188). The modern tarantati are musicians, artists, dancers and researchers of all ages and walks of life, often with unrelated full-time professions. For some the pizzica and other Salentine music are about amusement, a form of distraction to pass their summer nights following days spent on the beach, or just a passing fashion. For some it is a source of boredom, if not irritation, due to the endless repetition of the same songs. For a few it is more than that: a life philosophy, a message of love, a way of life.

Francesco Patruno (2003), meanwhile, has – on a less serious note – put together a list of categories of pizzica fans, emerging from what he calls 'the laws of the market that have cleared the piSSica through customs for the general public'.[14] For example:

> The Ubiquo (Ubiquitus Sempervirens Gramignicus): the nightmare par excellence. Ever since the piSSica phenomenon has reached such heights of diffusion, the UBIQUO is omnipresent and implacable. Anybody could be a ubiquitous piSSicophile, from your boss at work, to your neighbour, your newsagent, your friend, who, unexpectedly, from interests in entomology and butterflies coming from the mouth of the Orinoco has discovered that the piSSica pleases women, ergo it's a way of picking up a girl.

Patruno brilliantly shows how the use of the notion of tarantism and associated terms is motivated by many intertwined and contradictory facets: some broadcast via loudspeakers and every imaginable medium of communication, others restricted to closed circles or never even voiced.

'What does the pizzica mean to me?' Giorgio Di Lecce repeats my question to gather his thoughts. 'First, it is a form of self-expression. I am drawn to it because of my love for dance and theatre. Secondly, the pizzica provided a way of returning to my roots and of gaining knowledge of my own people. Thirdly, I found myself playing the tambourine for a tarantata in the chapel of Galatina from 1993 to 1995.'[15] Others, too, present the pizzica as a key to their origins, roots, grounding and identity. Director of the music group I Tamburellisti di Torrepaduli Pierpaolo De Giorgi asserts: 'Tarantism is about the consciousness of oneself. Tarantism, that's us, ourselves, as Apulia, as the Salento.'[16] Another passionate tambourine player reflects for a moment too: 'I'm not really sure why I'm attracted to this music and tarantism. Some things I just do because they feel right. I have always been very aware of the Church, its economic power and the influence it has on people and I've always tried to support those who are poor and powerless.'[17] A sense of empowerment emerges: music as rebellion, as a voice for the voiceless. One Salentine writer, meanwhile, speaks of his ambivalent feelings:

> I grew up in a small village with my grandmother. There were two tarantate who lived in her house; De Martino wrote about them. At first I was fascinated by this phenomenon. Then I hated it for many years, because I felt that those who were performing were putting on a show to gain attention. Then I became older and I began to realize the importance of this tradition.[18]

Meanwhile, music may speak for itself: on 14 February 2008, the funeral procession of Pino Zimba, much loved tambourine player, leader of the group Zimbaria and protagonist of the film Sangue Vivo, was accompanied by the rhythmic pounding of dozens of tambourines. This last passage of his life, too, was guided by the pizzica's beat. His body was laid to rest while the tarantula's music was evoked, linking the living and the dead.

Although performance contexts vary greatly, a continuum of neither exclusive nor exhaustive motives shapes the tarantula's music and dance: first, a small number of performers actively choose to draw on the system of tarantism to alleviate their suffering. They are unlikely to speak euphemistically about tarantism, as the current pizzica fashion occasionally risks doing. Secondly, others participate on stage, screen, canvas or paper, motivated by a desire to intellectually understand or artistically express past rituals. These participants, although aware of the distress underlying the lives of the tarantate and some nuovi tarantati, generally tend to close an eye to this aspect of suffering and may speak, instead, of tarantism as a feature that makes the Salento and its people unique. Thirdly, a large number of fans, including tourists, have been swept along by the recent boom in local music. With varying degrees of knowledge of the historical and contemporary meanings and experiences of the pizzica, their participation is motivated primarily by a desire for fun, pleasure and sensual gratification. Fourthly, there are those who find themselves attending a pizzica performance by chance, perhaps oblivious of its past links to tarantism, joining in as they would in any of the many entertainment programmes abounding during the summer season. Finally, some look on the tarantula's music and dance with suspicion and contempt, as one elderly woman explains: 'Especially the older women keep a stern face, saying that the devil is near. The older generations, like myself, are very aware of the force of the phenomenon of tarantism.'[19]

Clearly, today's tarantati are impossible to freeze into one or other fixed frame. Often self-definitions go hand in hand with definitions imposed by others and vary according to understandings of the tarantula's music and dance. It appears that, where an individual accepts this definition and others acknowledge it, a first step is taken to capturing the spider and its potential to promote well-being or discord: a glimpse of its outline as a shadow puppet made visible in conceptual and verbal form. How this form is then interpreted is tightly linked to broader conceptions of what is seen to make somebody ill or well.

Views on Venom: Interpreting the Spider's Bite

Inevitably, diagnoses of spider venoms depend on the cultural matrix of the viewer. Seventeenth-century views drew on the classical ideas of Hippocrates, Plato and Pythagoras and the 'humoral theory of correspondence' to explain the therapeutic potential of music: the four natural elements (earth, water, air and fire) linked to four bodily humours (blood, lymph, yellow and black bile) were seen to be rebalanced, in the case of affliction, by four basic corresponding musical modes (Mixolydian, Dorian, Lydian and Phrygian) (De Martino 2005: 223–36). Medical views of the same period, meanwhile, focused on the expulsion of venoms through perspiration (Katner 1956: 19–22).

Eighteenth-century religious discourses on the metaphysics of evil, instead, identified bodily impurities, such as spider poisoning, as signs of divine intervention: a punishment for sins committed, indications of St Paul's wrath or the devil's interference. Treatment involved seeking out the Apostle Paul and making offerings in exchange for grace, while recovery was equated with repentance and freedom from sin (Turner 1992). Enlightenment views, in the meantime, adopted Descartes's positivist approach, differentiating body and mind, and defining the tarantate's symptoms as psychological disorders, such as epilepsy, hysteria or schizophrenia (Di Mitri 2006). Treatment subsequently included electric shocks and pharmaceutical drugs.

Each rationalization was boosted by philosophical underpinnings, revealing the relativity of each view and the difficulty, if not impossibility, of pinpointing the multiple dimensions of experience and consciousness the term tarantism served to describe. Importantly, popular belief stated that the tarantate were not ill. There was nothing wrong with them. They were 'normal' people periodically subjected to the tarantula's whims.

Contemporary categorizations of Western medicine, meanwhile, entail risks of pathologizing the tarantate's condition. Robert Bartholomew (1994) contests widespread classifications of tarantism as one type of 'mass psychogenic illness', emphasizing the political advantages of making reference to the myth of the tarantula. A naturalistic explanation functioned to sanction personalistic explanations (Littlewood 1990: 313). In this way, non-Christian rituals could be pursued without risking persecution by the Church and, at the same time, 'revived the fledgling careers of many musicians restricted from performing by Church leaders' (Bartholomew 1994: 288).

Others have classified tarantism as a 'culture-bound syndrome' (Gentilcore 2000; Horden 2000), as an illness 'associated with culturally unique patterns of meaning superimposed on diseases that are universal' (Kleinman 1980: 77). This notion, however, easily serves as a standard label covering up culturally specific forms of expression, and attempts at defining it further (Simons and Hughes 1985) have revealed the danger of reducing it to one of various classical disorders of Western psychiatry, assuming that cultures variously impose meaning on universally identifiable biological conditions. Social anthropologist and psychiatrist Roland Littlewood (1990: 319) stresses:

> Western neuroses too are 'psychomedical' models of distress, and here the notion of 'disease' has a similar role to that of 'spirit possession' in less medicalized societies; both legitimize distress by removing personal responsibility while compelling others to act. Both express certain core social antagonisms in the personal situation of individuals and might perhaps be considered less as illnesses than as solutions.

It is useful, Littlewood adds (1990: 318), to consider such afflictions as part of a spectrum bridging the two poles of biomedical and sociological paradigms. Past cases of tarantism tended towards the sociological pole in their diagnosis. Precise biological causes may have been involved, but these appeared to act more as a final drop topping up an already full glass, as their direct relation to the tarantate's symptoms was not always clear. At times, an actual spider bite was recorded (De Martino 2005: 48). One of De Martino's informants was 'bitten' just after an operation in which her ovaries were removed, while another was suffering from an ear infection at the time of her affliction (ibid.: 56, 263).

Meanwhile, sociological paradigms were more easily identifiable in connection with the tarantula: bites generally happened in the summer; mainly women at specific life stages (especially puberty) were afflicted; several cases were often found in one family; tarantism was largely restricted to the region of Apulia; and, lastly, cures seemed to expire after one year (De Martino 2005: 25–27). Initial crises of tarantism commonly coincided with work – collecting peas, cutting vines, picking tobacco – or significant events such as driving over a snake (ibid.: 53), being bewitched by one (ibid.: 62) or inadvertent curses against St Paul (ibid.: 52).

Significant coincidences, concurrent with associations with a poisonous animal or the Apostle Paul, were generally established as causative incidents. Whatever the cause may have been and however this was interpreted, affliction by the 'mythic spider' appeared to involve extreme experiences, sharply cutting into and radically transforming the lives of those affected. As an aspect of the tangible and natural world, the tarantula was drawn upon to embody subjective dynamics, anchoring chaotic individual experience, materialized as poison, within the social and natural environment of the Salento.

But what acts as an explanatory framework now that the spiders are – apparently – gone from the fields? One modern tarantata explains:

> The tarantati of today are not ill. Suffering is involved, if you broaden its definition to include any state of unease, but De Martino's model is no longer valid for the new tarantati. I am not poor. I am not from a repressive society. I manage to have good relations with the people around me. And yet music touches me and I need to dance. The tarantati must be seen as depressed or melancholic, and the ritual and music are a way of providing a new consciousness, even if not on a rationally conscious level.[20]

'The affliction?' asks a young female dancer speaking of 'trance' experiences while dancing the pizzica. 'It's difficult: stagnant energy related to recent or ancient suffering? … For many years, I prohibited myself consciously or unconsciously from expressing things … from expressing myself in general … in order to accommodate other people's demands. The need to communicate, first and foremost, is not satisfied (now more than ever) … and the possibility to love and let yourself be loved' (Nacci 2004: 53–58). Maurizio Nocera confirms:

> Many individuals today actively choose to draw upon the system of tarantism to alleviate their suffering. There are many among the young who suffer in silence, but there are also many who are part of the world of tarantism. Do you know Giuseppe Marra? He frequently dances for three to four hours and, when you ask him why, he'll say that life isn't worth living.[21]

A deep-seated sensation of distress and a desire for meaning in life are evoked, calling for attention and leading Vittorio Lanternari (1995: 89) to identify a need

> to consider among the types of 'affliction' affecting the psychophysical organism of man, no longer only those illnesses catalogued in clinical repertoires, but also those 'states of being unwell' with no clinical denomination, that 'obscure affliction,' that indeterminable sense of emptiness, of a loss of points of reference and support, in sum, 'that suffering' which becomes concrete in definite and recognizable 'neuroses' or in particular psychosomatic syndromes.

We may ask to what extent such experiences of lacking roots and points of reference in life may relate to the 'crises of presence' De Martino (1956, 1961a) diagnosed among the tarantate. Such crises involved threatening situations in which individuals were unable to cope. Anthropologist Mariella Pandolfi (1990: 270) writes:

> To avoid this catastrophic outcome – the 'loss of presence' or failure of subjective identity in individuals and groups – people attempt by their choice of behaviour to manipulate psychic states through activities and practices which allow them to control the emergence of destructive impulses and to calm them, by channelling them into ritual performances, both individual and collective.

Inevitably, the notion of 'crises of presence' groups together a vast gamut of circumstances and experiences and, moreover, risks essentializing conceptions of the notion of presence itself. De

Martino himself (in Pandolfi 1990: 255) warns that 'there is no such thing as presence ... an inborn immediacy safe from all risk and incapable of ... history'.

We may query further to what extent social and political causes of affliction identified by De Martino, such as extreme poverty, harsh living conditions, excessive demands of labour, sexual repression or exclusion from public life, particularly of women, apply to the modern tarantati. The impacts of socio-economic development and the introduction of psychiatric care, identified as two key elements that have brought about the end of tarantism, are unlikely to safeguard against new problems that have emerged in the modern context of the Salento: high unemployment figures; large-scale emigration rupturing cultural and family ties; generational differences marking close-knit communities, to name just a few. Many women, moreover, have taken up professional careers, while continuing to bear the brunt of domestic tasks and the duties of caring for children and elderly family members (Goddard 1987, 1996; Goddard et al. 1996).

In these contexts, states of deep individual turmoil, reminiscent of De Martino's notion of 'crises of presence', may be triggered by a wide range of factors, including those with primarily biological foundations deflating the body's overall resistance, such as illness, accidents, operations, extreme physical exhaustion or persistent lack of sleep. Deeply emotional experiences such as childbirth or the traumatic loss of close personal relations may equally act as initial stimuli, as may the use of drugs. Such crises can, moreover, also be related to the lack of an explanatory framework, providing containment by pointing to customary problematic behaviour and how this may be dealt with.

Whereas in the past the model of tarantism provided a socially acknowledged existential framework, the modern tarantati may create or re-create their own model of this kind, engaging in a process of inscribing meaning, which inevitably risks incoherence and superficiality. This alerts us to Marianna Torgovnick's (1996: 176) warning about so-called New Age practices:

> On the basis of what I have seen, heard and read about the New Age, I believe that many of its participants are trapped in a rather moving contradiction. They adopt rituals and other aspects of cultures that depend fundamentally upon collective, communal experience – and sometimes on voiding or subordinating the autonomous self ... But New Agers almost invariably put these traditions and groups in the service of a thoroughly modern world view

that takes the self as a thing to be owned, cultivated and coddled – the veritable hub of the universe.

Such risks may apply equally, if not in an accentuated form, with the appropriation of the tarantula's music elsewhere, outside the Salento and Italy. There has, for instance, been a strong interest among Italo-American women in dancing the pizzica as a way of connecting with their Italian roots (Ciuffitelli 2005a).[22]

The controversial influence of Alessandra Belloni, New York-based percussionist and dancer, comes to mind. Her 'Rhythm is the Cure' workshops involve re-enactments of tarantism rituals and encourage women participants, often of Italian-American background, to self-identify as tarantate.[23] Belloni's work is generally viewed very critically among Salentines. Similarly, the case of a young Frenchwoman, seen to be a tarantata in need of ritual music by a number of Salentine musicians who played for her in a series of encounters during the 2000 summer, evoked strong criticism, particularly among women, regarding the manipulation of the tradition of tarantism and the musicians involved.[24]

Although the tarantula's music and dance are, generally speaking, performed today in contexts that do not re-create a feasible milieu in which those afflicted can rely on the social support of a group to express and process their afflictions, the experiences of Ada, Tanya and others nevertheless present examples of how these performance practices indicated one possible way out, allowing – to various degrees – for a recovery of a sense of balance within the individual and within their larger network of relations.

These examples stress not only the risks involved in re-appropriating perceived healing practices, both in the area of their apparent origins or elsewhere, but also how such processes of re-appropriation inevitably depend on the availability of options seen to be beneficial – and acceptable – to the recovery of well-being.

Tarantula Alternatives: Choosing Treatment Options

In the Salento, therapeutic options have multiplied. What did people do when they were ill in the past? 'They died!' a woman in her eighties told me, without any thought to my question or emotion to match her response.[25] Illness categories have also proliferated. 'There are a lot more illnesses today,' says another elderly woman. 'Everyone immediately goes to the doctor. I myself only take something for my blood pressure. Illnesses in the past were cured with the available means. Coffee was used when someone fainted. Then it was a luxury. Today, even I have coffee every morning.'[26] A comparative look at past and present means of treatment shows that, although facilities have greatly changed and expanded, their application depended and depends on a process of negotiating choices.

In earlier decades, hospitals were non-existent or kilometres away. Transport problems and expense stood in the way of consulting medical staff. Psychiatry, in particular, was never an option until some decades ago. Other specialists, including priests, doctors, traditional practitioners known as *macare* and snake-handling *sanpaolari*, were resorted to, as tarantism rituals were one alternative in a spectrum of treatment options within broader magico-religious belief systems (De Martino 1960; Gentilcore 1992, 1998).[27] Historical documents, meanwhile, reveal a broad gamut of cures applied to cases of tarantism beyond the use of music and dance.[28]

The English traveller George Berkeley (1717) tells how some tarantate were administered a concoction of wine prepared with a fossilized snake-tongue after their third day of dancing. The *serparo*, or snake-handler, once widespread in Apulia, could offer related treatments. His expertise was in drawing poison out of wounds using conjurations and such verbal incantations (Chiaia 1887; Turchini 1987: 165) as the prayer formula 'Io ti esorcizzo da ogni morso' (I exorcize you of every bite), apparently dating back to the ninth or tenth century (Di Mitri 1995: 222). For the tarantate such formulas were at times combined with the drawing of a cross above the bite mark and the drinking of water from the holy well in Galatina (Caputo 1741: 228). The tarantula's victims may also have consulted a *macara*, with expertise in magical affairs, to assess whether causes such as the 'evil eye' were at stake. One case from 1627, recorded by the ecclesiastical tribunal, reveals how a woman named Catarina Palazzo treated a tarantata with a conjuration, incense, sacred water and by touching painful body parts with her prescriptive books (Tamblé 2000: 106).

Catholicism provided further options for relief. Exorcist priests were conferred with to identify whether the devil's influence was at hand and sanctuaries of saints credited with healing powers were visited.[29] In the Salento itself, the case of St Donatus shows that tarantism was only one of various related phenomena that provided a therapeutic option in the face of hardship and suffering. During his lifetime, legend goes, St Donatus cured those possessed by the devil, and epilepsy became known as *il male di San Donato*, St Donatus's illness, or *il morbo sacro*, the sacred disease. On his feast day, 7 August, pilgrims still come to his chapel in the town of Montesano Salentino. In 1998, when I attended this festival, hundreds of devotees came to say their prayers and leave offerings of money. Numerous 100,000 lire[30] notes decorated the saint's statue and one elderly female informant told of inexplicable things she had seen, reminiscent of the 'miraculous' deeds attributed to the tarantate at Galatina: 'In the past, the number of devotees coming here was much greater: everyone afflicted by St Donatus's illness came. You recognized them because they jerked their limbs all over the place. I remember seeing one woman, dressed all in white, dancing on top of the saint's statue. It seems impossible, but I saw it with my own eyes.'[31]

Similarly, the opinion of doctors, when available, was sought out by the tarantate, although their symptoms often escaped diagnostic categories. 'The doctors didn't find anything wrong with me,' the tarantato Francesco Greco explained. 'They say that we are mad and putting on a show, because our bodies are essentially healthy.'[32] In more recent decades, many tarantate were taken to psychiatric specialists.

What options of treatment and support, meanwhile, cater to those who define themselves as nuovi tarantati in relation to experiences of affliction in the contemporary Salento? Biomedical practitioners, especially those working in the fields of psychiatry and psychology, may be a key source of reference, although the stigma associated with mental health care may inhibit many from seeking their help. Ada, who danced for the TV cameras in June 2001, tells of undergoing psychoanalysis but eventually abandoning this while continuing to dance. Other factors will have played their part, but clearly the tarantula's music and dance provided a perceived benefit not accessible through conventional health care. Complementary medicine, including music or art therapies, has been a little-known alternative until recently.[33] Now these professions are growing, as art therapy courses, homeopathy schools and other forms of complementary medicine of various types and degrees of professionalism proliferate.[34]

However, widespread public opinion in the Salento tends to remain critical towards complementary medical treatments available, as techniques and explanatory models may be taken from non-Western contexts, rendering them alien to potential clients (Lüdtke 2003). Rita Cappello, music therapist at the rehabilitation clinic Casa di Cura 'Villa Verde' in Lecce, explains that one of the greatest difficulties she faces with music therapy patients is a resistance to play, expressed in such defensive reactions as: 'I'm no longer at the age to play around or sing!'[35] Play and artistic expression are rarely recognized as methodologies with therapeutic potential.

Clearly, views of treatment options, forged largely by a widespread familiarity with biomedicine, may not correspond with the practices proposed. An extreme example of this emerged in a 1999 music therapy workshop I attended near Lecce. This included the use of an Australian didgeridoo to show how acoustic vibrations directed at different body parts could 'stimulate specific organs'. One participant later described this event as bringing up associations of satanic reunions.[36] Such issues as the use of out-of-context practices; the commercial exploitation of what Lanternari (2000: 133) calls 'multinational religious industries'; or the exaltation of individual development in preference to communal and social welfare are all familiar criticisms levelled at the New Age movement. All of these may act as obstacles to those in search of therapeutic alternatives.

Similar discrepancies in belief and practice may prevent many who live in the Salento today from considering 'traditional practitioners' as a therapeutic option.[37] I talked to one such practitioner who treated a variety of ailments, including burns, benign tumours and dislocations, but when asked about tarantism vehemently insisted that these were practices of the devil.[38] Religious healers practising within the context of Catholicism may be another point of reference, with a small number of priests apparently still performing exorcisms and saints attributed with healing qualities being central in this respect. Votive offerings present another socially condoned option of religious healing practices available to devotees. Nevertheless, rejection of the Catholic Church at large, especially among younger generations, may discourage the modern tarantati from considering this option.

It becomes clear that an alternative route to well-being, possibly tucked away within the rave-like, delirious movement of the pizzica, is welcome to many. The pizzica is socially accepted, if not glorified, and, rather than excluding and stigmatizing, draws participants into its circle, into the limelight. Something more than celebrity is at stake, pointing to the need for careful, case-by-case consideration of past and present spider dances.

A first step may be taken by comparing the case of the modern tarantata Ada Metafune with that of Maria of Nardò, a tarantata in the historical sense of the term. Whereas individuals afflicted by the tarantula in the past were likely to be assigned their role as tarantate by others and through the process of undergoing rituals of tarantism, Ada's view of herself as a modern tarantata appears to be self-assigned, even if in relation to the re-valorization of the pizzica in the Salento and elsewhere. Moreover, for the tarantate of yesteryear, music was deliberately applied for healing within the context of an acknowledged belief system and considered to be the only way out. Meanwhile, Ada retrospectively views her involvement in the music and dance of the pizzica as curative, in the light of her own acquaintance with therapeutic alternatives such as psychoanalysis. Likewise, past performances were determined by a ritual context focused on the symbolic complex of the tarantula spider, whereas Ada has re-enacted this ritual on many occasions for theatrical purposes or television cameras and her motivations for doing so may be questioned. Many tarantate in the past, too, were accused of putting on a show. Such persisting questions of authenticity may become secondary, however, if we acknowledge that the impacts of cultural performances, even if staged, may be real in their effects on a level of experience and, moreover, that the healing power of the pizzica was acknowledged in the past, not only in ritual performances, but equally in its performances on manifold festive occasions (Lüdtke 2005a).

Despite major discrepancies between the performance contexts of the tarantate and the neo-tarantati, the dances of both must be considered in relation to the negotiative processes involved, bringing into play individual, social and political aspects of recovering well-being. Performances may transfix participants by imposing out-of-context beliefs and practices. At the same time, they may also provide a way of integrating and making sense of difficult experiences in the lives of those seen to be transfixed by the tarantula.

Notes

1. Gallipoli, 12 June 1999.
2. Galatina, 29 June 1998.
3. Soleto, 4 April 1998.
4. Lecce, 4 December 1997.
5. Lecce, 24 November 1997.
6. Lecce, 2 February 1998.
7. 'The term *widow* spider originated from the idea that the females devour the males after, or during, mating. This mate devouring behaviour is somewhat a myth; while it may occur in captive situations, where the male cannot escape, it is uncommon in the field.' Retrieved on 19 July 2007 from http://www.srv.net /~dkv/hobospider/widows.html.
8. Personal communication.
9. I thank Damian Walter for bringing these links to my attention.
10. Lecce, 14 February 1998.
11. Scorrano, 12 July 1999.
12. Teatro Paisiello, Lecce, 15 May 1998.
13. Maurizio Nocera (2005: 10) identifies *tarantati*: 'those who feel the suffering of the bite or re-bite for having entered into competition with a divinity (the Greek Athena, the Latin Minerva, the Christian St Paul), which "punishes" them by inflicting their body with possession by the spider'; *attarantati*: 'those who simulate the tarantate in spectacularized and dramaticized theatrical scenes'; and *attarantanti*: 'intellectuals (though not alone) who, for reasons of study or other particular interests, were or are interested in this phenomenon, and as a result remain strongly influenced up to the point of taking on related forms of behaviour.'
14. Patruno's choice to use the double 's' rather than double 'z' spelling here is intentional. Perhaps a deliberate hint at 'taking the piss' in the sense of making fun of or ridiculing someone or something?
15. Lecce, 20 February 1998.
16. Galatina, 29 June 1999.
17. Tricase, 27 November 1997.
18. Lecce, 4 December 1997.
19. Lecce, 24 November 1997.
20. Lecce, 14 February 1998.
21. Lecce, 1 April 2006.
22. See the video *Pizzica with a New York Accent* (Ciuffitelli 2005b).
23. Italian-American cultural project manager Mary Ciuffitelli has looked into Belloni's influence in more detail (Ciuffitelli 2005a), as has Italian scholar and singer Laura Biagi (Biagi 2004).
24. See Collu (2005: 59–73) for a description of this case.
25. Montesano, 16 November 1997.

26. Tricase, 2 May 1998.

27. The dialect term *macara* or *maciara* is translated as *strega* in Italian, meaning witch or sorceress (Rohlfs 1956–1961). The *sanpaolari*, meanwhile, were seen to be inheritors of St Paul's healing powers, and were often viewed as charlatans tainting the reputation of those with honest motivations (Turchini 1987; Montinaro 1996). Their antidotes included holy water and earth, *la terra di San Paolo*, taken from St Paul's grotto in Malta and used to sculpt medals, amulets, vases, cups, tablets or model statues of the apostle. Fossilized serpent teeth or tongues, *glossopietre* or *lingue di San Paolo*, of Maltese origin were also part of their remedy kit.

28. Remedies suggested for cases of tarantism include: 'a prescription containing twenty-four herbs and spices' (Caputo 1741: 133); *Alexipharmaca*, a treatise dealing with poisons and their antidotes (Sigerist 1948: 110); healing saliva (Vallone 2004); crushed garlic mixed with treacle spread onto the bite to neutralize the poison; diaphoretics (administered to produce perspiration); draughts of lemon rind, parsley, mint, wild thyme and berries; alcohol mixed with treacle or rosemary (Russell 1979: 411–14). Treatment techniques involved: scarification, cupping and cauterization (Sigerist 1948: 110); *la cura del forno caldo*, the warm oven cure (Vandenbroeck 1997: 101; De Martino 2005: 215); blistering of feet and bathing in warm water; hydrotherapy; the use of cloths warmed and moistened in wine and wrapped around the naked body; bandaging of the bite with a ligature (Russell 1979: 411–14).

29. The sanctuary of San Cosimo della Macchia just south of Oria, attracting numerous pilgrims and holding an enormous display of votive offerings, still stands as a contemporary shrine dedicated to St Cosmas, one of the key healers in the Catholic tradition.

30. The approximate equivalent of 52.00 euros (using the conversion rate of 1,936.27 lire to one euro from 1 January 2002, when the euro was first introduced).

31. Montesano, 6 August 1998.

32. 11 August 1999.

33. Between 1997 and 1999, I followed the work of Rita Cappello and her group of music and art therapists, Musicarte, working with the method *la globalità dei linguaggi* (Guerra-Lisi 1987), who were very much pioneering this work at the time.

34. Giuliano Capani's (2004) film *Un ritmo per l'anima: tarantismo e terapie naturali*, A Rhythm for the Soul: Tarantism and Natural Therapies, is a recent cinematographic document comparing and contrasting tarantism with present treatment and meditation practices involving rhythmic interaction.

35. Lecce, 21 July 1999.

36. Lecce, 20 July 1999.

37. I use this term to refer to practitioners using traditional healing modalities generally including herbal treatment and spiritual care.

38. Lucugnano, 13 May 1998.

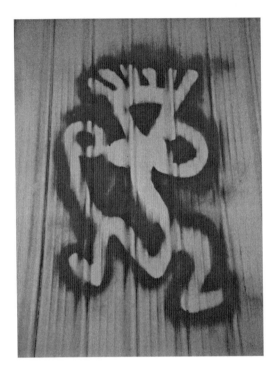

Fig. 7.1 Graffiti painting of the 'dancing god', Porto Badisco, July 1998 (photo: Karen Lüdtke).

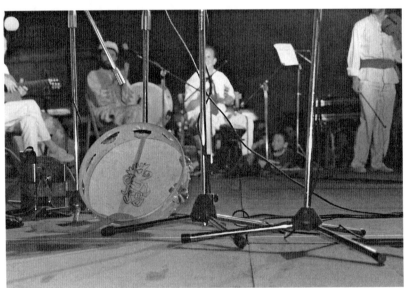

Fig. 7.2 The 'dancing god' on stage on a tambourine skin during a concert of the group Arakne Mediterranea, Galatina, 29 June 1999 (photo: Karen Lüdtke).

Chapter 7
Tarantula Threads and Showbiz Airs: Fine-tuning Performances

> Two people dancing in the centre of a circle
> are like a fire heating everyone looking on.
>
> Tambourine player, Ostuni, 21 May 1998

A girl no more than ten years old writhes on a white sheet. A young woman circles its perimeter, waving a red scarf at her in an elegantly tamed bullfighting fashion. It is a mild summer night in September 1999 and a crowd has gathered in the town of Casarano for a concert of the Alla Bua. The musicians had announced the young dancer's request to repeat a piece rehearsed for her school performance. One of them kneels close to the dancer on the tarmac sports pitch, the concert venue, beating a large, cymbal-less tambourine (a 'shamanic drum', as he specifies) with a wooden drumstick, and spectators enclose the performance space.

The girl dancer, dressed in a white dress and white sandals, moves rhythmically, rolling back and forth across the bleached linen sheet before coming to her feet to dance steps of the pizzica within the sheet's contours. Eventually, she collapses gently to the ground only to repeat this sequence several times until the musicians come to the end of their piece. Flashes of Maria of Nardò's performance filmed in 1959 (Carpitella 1960) come to mind, with this perfect rendition of the main dance cycles of tarantism rituals as described by De Martino. The applause is enthusiastic. Clearly, it appears, this is what parents, schoolteachers and other onlookers want to see: a performance infused with the aesthetic criteria of a school ballet production; a depiction of the socially desired grace and gentleness of a well-brought-up young girl; an enactment of femininity as docile and compliant, all the more pleasing when perceived as the spontaneous wish of a young community member wanting to show and share what she has learnt.

Technically, a ritual of tarantism has been re-enacted. Yet I am left with the sense of an empty shell of reproduced movements. On the level of performative expressivity, there was little, if any, connection with the tarantate's dance of bygone years. There was no hint of the crises and conflicts women (and men) conveyed through this ritual, no glimpse of the aggression and transgressive eroticism breaking social and sexual norms of the time. Considering this disjuncture, what tools can be applied to compare what was a ritual embedded within a magico-religious belief system and what is predominantly a show or (well-dusted) museum piece?

A focus on four key aspects: places, times, props (or performative devices) and techniques brings to the fore the tangible – musical and choreographic – aspects of performances, as well as principal factors seen to promote efficacy.[1] Like the musicians of the tarantate, today's musicians have to 'tune in' to a place and its people, finding the rhythms that stir, excite and stimulate. This relies on a maximum number of participants agreeing to collaborate in the collectively acknowledged reality and rules of a performance. No single element determines success. Instead, it is the appropriate combination of various elements that brings out 'the magic' people marvel at. Such appropriateness relies on specific knowledge acquired through experience, and is constantly open to negotiation and change.

Existing studies in anthropology and performance provide a valuable backdrop here. Theatre scholars searching for tools to understand performance in Western contexts have always been concerned with theatre's relation to the intangible spheres of human existence, the metaphysical, invisible, supernatural, ethical or holy (Artaud 1958; Brecht 1964; Grotowski 1976; Stanislavski 1980a, b, 1981; Brook 1998; Barba 2001). Their work highlights the social and potentially spiritual and moral side of theatrical performance, suggesting parallels to religious or ritual practice. Anthropologists, in turn, have aimed at overcoming simplistic distinctions between theatre and ritual, as well as ethnocentric interpretations of performance, by taking culturally specific contexts into account (Grotowski 1976; Beattie 1977; V. Turner 1982; Schechner 1988, 2002; Schieffelin 1996). This has brought to the fore the importance of performance in regard to other human institutions or social constructions, such as religion, politics, gender or ethnicity.

A shift in the consideration of dramatic practices, from being viewed 'largely in terms of structures of representations to being seen as processes of practice and performance' (Schieffelin 1996: 59), has placed attention on the socially and individually constructed nature of such practices. Ethnomusicologists and dance ethnologists (Williams 1991; Stokes 1994; Reed 1998; Buckland 1999, 2006; Farnell 1999; Guss 2000; Kaeppler 2000; Thomas 2003; Peterson Royce 2004; Post 2006) have contributed fundamentally to such an understanding of performance as a 'vital form of social creativity' (Stokes 1994: 24) able to generate, negotiate and control meanings and experiences; as intrinsically political and paradoxical (Cohen 1993); and as 'part of the very construction and interpretation of social and conceptual relationships and processes' (Seeger 1987: xiv).

Without dismissing major differences, the conceptual gulf between the notions of theatre and ritual becomes less straightforward when considering the phenomenological level of experience:

> 'Performances – whether ritual or dramatic – create and make present realities vivid enough to beguile, amuse or terrify. They alter moods, attitudes, social states and states of mind. Unlike texts, however, they are ephemeral; they create their effects and then are gone, leaving their reverberations (fresh insights, reconstituted selves, new statuses, altered realities) behind them.' (Schieffelin 1996: 59)

Moreover, as David Parkin (1996: xxi) writes: 'Cultural performance is real in its effects but, because imagined, gives its creators and their audiences a freedom of invention and interpretation that does not exist with regard to structured or positive reality.' Performances, whether theatre or ritual, become an experimental platform exposing participants to new roles and experiences, providing a means of contesting, manipulating and creating social constructions of the self, others and the world around.

With a focus on the processual nature of performance practices, how did and does the Italian spider's dance beguile, amuse or terrify? What alternative realities were and are created? Perceptions of performative efficacy, and how this is negotiated, provide a helpful guideline. A look at places that characterize first past and then present dances posits an initial step to explore what factors may be variously seen to distinguish a hit from a flop.

Spider Sites: Performance Places

'Once we followed a tarantata down this road playing our instruments. She was crawling on her stomach imitating the serpent that had bitten her,' explained Luigi Stifani, well-known violinist of the tarantate, as we walked through his hometown of Nardò, towards his barber's shop.[2] On the front door, there was a sign reading *Studio di cultura sul tarantolismo* marking this salon, too, with the spider's imprint.[3]

Up until De Martino's research in 1959, public spaces, village squares, streets or courtyards and, arguably, even churches became stages for the tarantate's rituals, as did private spheres, closed homes and secluded bedrooms. Historically, picturesque natural sites were favourite choices: fields, country roads and shady spots abundant in vegetation and water (De Martino 2005: 87). At first glance, it appears that almost any spot could be carved into a stage. However, a location's association with the initial 'bite' or 'crisis' most frequently determined decisions.

Today, the chapel and grotto of St Paul in Galatina and Giurdignano remain two publicly accessible sites evoking the tarantula.[4] Although many are oblivious of these places, they stand as testimony to powerful tensions between the Catholic Church and popular religious or spiritual needs. Although long since deconsecrated officially, devotees continue to come here and others insist that they are preserved.[5]

Early manuscripts and maps, meanwhile, conflated the tarantula spider with the Salento or Apulia as a whole. European travellers documented these practices with disbelief and suspicion (Boyle 1685; Burney 1771; Swinburne 1783), often taking them as proof of the ignorance and backwardness of southern Italy at large.[6] Burney presents scientific experiments disclaiming the views of believers: 'Dr. Cirillo assured me that he had never been able to provoke that tarantula either to bite himself or others upon whom he had repeatedly tried the experiment. However, the whole is so thoroughly believed by some innocent people in the country' (1771: 313). He adds an apologetic footnote in the name of scientific progress: 'This account may perhaps diminish the honour of music, by augmenting the number of sceptics, as to its *miraculous powers*; yet truth requires it should be given' (ibid.).

It was also often claimed that the tarantula's bite was harmless beyond Apulian borders and poisonous only to those of Apulian origin.

Other southern Italian case studies contradict these views (Pitré 1894; Zanetti 1978; Rossi 1991), but the concentration of tarantism in Italy's heel cannot be explained as mere coincidence. De Martino tells of a Sicilian woman who became a tarantata after moving to the Salento and of a young Salentine who apparently continued to perform tarantism rituals while committed to military service in northern Italy (2005: 65). Others felt the tarantula's bite as they settled back in the Salento after years of working abroad (Miscuglio et al. 1981; Mingozzi 1982). Spider threads inevitably reached beyond Apulian ground and infiltrated foreign bloodstreams, but always maintained conceptual connections with their perceived southern Italian source.

The region of Apulia was also seen as inseparable from the indigenous music and dance of the tarantella. Dancing in the contexts of merrymaking at weddings, festivals and other social occasions is likely to have provided a training ground for ritual choreographies. 'The old musicians', one Salentine musician in his fifties confirms, 'all have a sensitivity for places.'[7]

> Tarantism is something that leads you to feel things, to feel the air, the particles which vibrate, such as the wind, for instance. The wind has a sound. To me, for example, it communicates a great number of things. To play the pizzica well you need a lot of training, a lot of resistance, because you begin to feel well only after three to four hours of playing. That's when energy begins to circulate and there's resonance. And then there are many other things, you travel, you see everything. The sound becomes one, until you don't feel anything any more, and you begin to see everything from above; these things are all part of the experiences you have.[8]

The harsh reality of bygone training contexts was seen to further this ability. Luigi Toma tells how he learnt in the *ronde*, or circles, of Torrepaduli: 'if you didn't keep in time with a circle, you were thrown out with a kick – bam! Certain times were established. People from each town kept to specific rhythms and to specific people. If you entered their circle and wanted to play but at a certain point no longer kept up, they threw you out!'[9] Another musician adds:

> I began playing when I was a child. At the popular festivals you played non-stop from evening until morning. There were no breaks for a minimum of eight to nine hours. This gives you the capacity to play when you grow up. The organism, the body, is made for playing. Now this isn't the case any more. The young people no longer manage to do this, they don't have the physical resistance.[10]

Playing the pizzica demanded physical endurance and stamina, which past generations are likely to have gained through hard manual labour as well as long hours of music making and dancing. However, not everyone played and danced. One elderly woman in her eighties emphasized that there was no time between work in the fields, factories and home.[11]

Just as skills in music making and dancing were passed down the generations, cases of affliction often predominated in a single family, as if inherited or acquired through the process of socialization. Difficult living conditions and problematic relationships were perpetuated, as was a familiarity with devices – both technical and conceptual – required to enact rituals. In this sense, the actual process of growing up in the Salentine environment sculpted individuals, both physically and perceptually, to be able to perform if and when the need arose. Moreover, as Damian Walter points out: 'If the Salentine peninsula was as harsh as it seemed to be – and if tarantism further expressed peasant women's frustrated sexuality and anxieties about fertility (deaths of young children, etc.) – then it seems possible that tarantism's association with "naturally picturesque sites" reflects a broader concern with the natural rhythms and fecundity of the landscape itself.'[12]

Others have similarly stressed the links between ritual procedures and natural surroundings, as well as working life. A tambourine player from Ostuni suggests a link between the rhythm of the pizzica and the song of the *cinciarella* (blue tit), a migratory bird found in southern Italy, marked by a lively 'tee, tee, tee' followed by a scolding 'chirr'.[13] I have not heard others make this connection, although some identified animal behaviour in dance moves. One dancer showed me how a male performer might imitate a cockerel, with a stretched-out hand quivering above his forehead, or a bee or serpent moving to sting or bite: with the index and middle fingers curved slightly downwards to simulate a poisonous needle or tongue, the male dancer approaches his female partner and, using his fingers to draw figures of eight in the air in front of her face and body, suddenly launches forward, stings, so to speak, without touching and retreats immediately while closing his outstretched fingers into a fist, as if to retrieve and carry away some invisible essence.[14]

Another musician adds that everyday working life may have provided further inspiration, as his hands stretch upwards to illustrate the motions of picking fruit or vine twigs.[15] The tambourine, the musicians'

164

key prop, provides a further link to work. It is made of animal skin (usually goat or cow hide) stretched over a circular wooden frame to which metal cymbals are attached. This frame was, and to a lesser extent is, also used by artisans to make work tools: covered with a metal netting or pierced animal skin it becomes a *farnaru* (sieve), used with rhythmic movements to sift flour. Associations with other forms of daily work come to mind, raising questions about the rhythmic nature of this work (and its daily tedium) in relation to the rhythms of dancing and playing. The crafts of weaving or spinning, in particular (central to the legend of Arachne), played a prime role in women's tasks in bygone days, creating analogies to the weaving of relationships on a social level and the spinning of fate – by the three Fates or goddess Aphrodite in Greek mythology, for example – on a cosmic level (Kinsley 1995: 193–94).

In twenty-first-century Italy, meanwhile, spider webs continue to merge with Salentine (as well as Apulian) longitudes and latitudes. Assertions of local identities foster views of this region as home to the unique tradition of tarantism (Apolito 2000). In 2000, the local tourist board's postcards, decked with a tambourine and a couple dancing the pizzica, proclaimed the Salento as: 'Aperto tutto l'anno' (Open all year round) [see Fig. 4.1]. The music and dance of the tarantula make front-page material, attracting thousands to this region. An influx of one hundred thousand tourists was estimated solely in the period around the 2005 Notte della Taranta (Maruccio 2005). Most come for the summer concerts, but have no illusions of (or desire for) stumbling across a healing ritual of bygone days. Yet claims that these may persist at sites hidden in the Salentine countryside create expectation (Santoro 1982: 75). Any spot on the peninsula might still be a sacred stage for the tarantula: perhaps insider knowledge, not kept as secret as it could be, creates a halo of mystery and, in any case, good publicity.

Village squares, closed-off crossroads, seaside promenades and countryside venues are preferred contemporary showcases for the tarantula's music and dance. Abandoned farmhouses or rural chapels, widespread in the Salento, are other favourite sites. With generators fuelling light bulbs and loudspeakers and traffic signs attracting and directing crowds, deserted and silent places become temporarily infused with life. Props – such as flames lining the track leading to a performance or flickering on buildings around a stage – set the scene and mark places as out of the ordinary.

Although brightly spotlighted public stages with powerful hi-fi systems, including discothèques (Bruno 1999; Maruccio 1999), rule the popular music and dance scene, more enclosed, private spheres and celebrations also frequently host the pizzica. Birthday parties and other social gatherings held in the privacy of homes are welcome excuses to pull out the tambourine. The Pizzeria Lu Puzzu in the *Griko* town of Sternatia has become famous for its Tuesday-night pizzica sessions staged among the restaurant tables as an after-dinner digestive. Similarly, in autumn 2002, the Thurn und Taxis Pub in Lecce promoted weekly pizzica jam sessions. In verbal rather than musical form, conferences, book presentations and theatre productions bring the tarantula alive, on both outdoor and indoor stages. Art exhibitions and film productions throw its sounds and images onto canvas screens in galleries, cultural associations and cinemas, while workshops introduce it to school syllabuses and university auditoriums.

Students are animated to rediscover their roots, while tourists are invited to explore the exotic. The Salentine peninsula collapses into the tarantula as a poster promoting the 2004–05 season of the Lecce football team shows. Above the slogan *Terra di Serie A*, League A Country, a spider crawls over Italy's heel painted in the team's red and yellow colours, ironically precisely those that were seen to most affect the tarantate of the past. Far from soccer stadiums, a select number of intellectually inspired friends and followers of the late Salentine poet and artist Antonio Verri have identified certain sites in the Salentine countryside as representative of the contemporary world of tarantism, sites that express the *sibilo lungo* or deep murmur.[16] Although perhaps previously irrelevant to the tarantate, these landmarks – St Paul's grotto in Giurdignano, the Porto Badisco cave paintings, Torre St Emiliano [see Figs 0.3 and 3.1–3.3] and others – have acquired contemporary meanings through the historical, religious or mystical import assigned to them (Chiriatti 1995; Lüdtke 2002). They are sites of devotion where the much-used phrase *la mia terra* – my homeland, my earth, my roots – appears condensed into material form, instilling and reconfirming an awareness of the self as linked to the Salentine territory, especially when infused with music making and dancing. Fernando Bevilacqua put it this way: 'There are certain places where I need to go during the year. It's like an exorcism, as if to wish myself to continue to live.'[17]

People and places conceptually shape each other. The tarantula becomes a matrix for the Salento and its people and vice versa. Each one creates and moulds the other. Meanings are projected onto a site, like a movie onto a screen, and the greater the sense of reality of this projection the greater the perceived efficacy of the performance. Anyone doubting, questioning or criticizing bursts this bubble of projection, cutting through the movie screen. With the Church's attempts to prohibit tarantism rituals, the tarantate increasingly performed behind locked doors. Today, too, success is jeopardized if the associations ascribed to a place deviate from those ascribed to a performance. Likewise, performance times play a key role in determining success.

Spider Schedules: Performance Times

The tarantula's venom could strike at any time, day or night, and in any season of the year. However, initial crises coincided mostly with the hot summer months, under the auspices of the burning sun. Everyday life was at its harshest and the spider abundant in the fields. This was also the time of St Paul's festival. The anniversary of a first bite often provoked crises anew, as did other festive or social events. States of emergency could be treated at any time, but the hottest part of the day was seen as most conducive to recovery. Francesco Greco, who danced to the tunes of the tarantula in the 1960s, confirms this: 'The musicians came around 11 a.m., because that was the time, more or less, when this animal started to show its effects, the hot hours, from 11 a.m. to 2 p.m.. Those were the three peak hours.'[18] Sweating was most profuse then, facilitating – as was believed – the expulsion of the spider's venom.

Ritual phases lasted ten to fifteen minutes on average, followed by short breaks of another ten minutes or so. Generally, recovery required a minimum of three to four days of dancing, with rests at night-time. Moreover, De Martino was told, St Paul gave his grace either at 12 noon, 1 p.m., 3 p.m. or 5 p.m. (2005: 42). Although these claims are hard to follow up, rituals were wrapped into the sun's twenty-four-hour cycle and annual rhythm: when the sun was at its highest and most intense, the tarantula's bite was most profuse and its dance likely to be most efficient. It also generally hit at specific points in a life cycle, most often during puberty or early adulthood, or in moments of major transitions, such as childbirth, marriage or loss of a spouse (De Martino 2005: 83). While some tarantate never repeated their initial performance, others, like Evelina, continued to do so for over half a century on every anniversary of their 'initial bite'.

Nowadays, meanwhile, the pizzica escapes the burning sun, as pleasantly air-conditioned summer nights are its main showcase. Village festivals and *sagre*, food fairs, have in recent years rarely been complete or truly traditional, so to speak, without this music's stamp. Although summer nights still hold the strongest spell, the pizzica may heat up any night of the year. The winter bonfire festival of St Anthony, for instance, celebrated in the small suburb of Villa Convento on 22 January 2005, was set to its rhythms. Although just a small gathering with a few sausage and chestnut stands, the pizzica was not missing.

While seasonal and religious cycles still influence the tarantula's beat, other cycles equally hold it in their grip. In spring 1998, during the local election campaign for Lecce's new mayor, pizzica concerts followed political speeches of all inclinations: spider music turned into political catchphrase and voting trigger. Meanwhile, annual events, such as the Night of the Tarantula or the Pizzicata Festival,[19] follow the examples of major world music initiatives counting on the perennial pilgrimage of fans. Workshops and seminars organized by schools or the University of Lecce offer an intellectual or artistic tone according to the academic calendar. Likewise, my own neighbourhood in Lecce became the inadvertent audience to a didgeridoo, ringing out through the open balcony doors of a nearby flat, in tune to pizzica songs on summer nights in 2007.

Such one-off happenings may have few immediately evident links to broader temporal patterns anchoring these events within the rhythms of daily life. Moreover, although the tarantula's music and dance come alive mostly at night, no specific hours can be allocated to their performances. Where events mix verbal, visual and musico-choreographic elements, a temporal hierarchy emerges: lectures and films, representing the tarantula's case in words, images and recordings, set the scene and mood, creating a gradual build-up to the actual music making and dancing. Finally, a few hard-core performers often hang around after the official performance is over and microphones have been unplugged. Spontaneous circles, at times lasting into the early morning hours, provide time to improvise and unwind.

When a show, whether of past or contemporary spider dances, is embedded into larger acknowledged social and natural cycles, participation is legitimized and encouraged. Through correspondence and repetition it is anchored into the passage of time, as defined by everyday life. In cases of tarantism, symptoms often involved responses of withdrawal from temporally specific circumstances, a means of periodically propelling individuals into a sphere that was free from the influence of cyclical patterns and the hardships these may have entailed. Rituals, meanwhile, could guide the individual within this sphere through the imposition of performative rhythms rooted in the socio-natural rhythms of daily life, thereby aiming to draw the individual's sensory perception outwards and to coax the afflicted back into the present time and place. In modern circumstances, performances may still be linked to seasonal and religious cycles, but detachment from these cycles – be it, for instance, through air-conditioned and centrally heated lives or a lack of common belief systems – gives more credit to other cycles, such as those of commerce, politics and tourism, often boasting their closeness to nature and the authentic past as a catchphrase.

Respecting the cyclical process of a performance may be seen to boost efficacy. Rituals were characterized by phases of preparation, exploration, climax and repose. Staged shows equally benefit from a gradual build-up of rhythm and atmosphere, a variable period of intense playing, and an improvised and more laid-back time to finish off, without amplifications or schedule of any kind. Accordingly, participants are required to surrender to the continuity and unity of the performance rhythms for efficacy to take its course. This requires being sensitive not only to places and times but also to the props and techniques engaged with.

Tarantula Threads: Past Props and Techniques

'If you didn't find the tarantula's thread,' an elderly tarantato from the town of Acaya explained (Di Lecce 1994: 191), 'they didn't manage to dance, they didn't manage to move.' *Il filo della taranta*, the thread

169

of the tarantula, had to be found: that stimulus, be it a rhythm, melody, colour, image, scent or object, which would instigate the bitten woman (or man) to react and, most importantly, to dance. *I tempi giusti*, the 'right' tempo or rhythms, had to be established in order to provoke an irresistible urge to dance. Musical exploration aimed at finding a trigger, an emotional button that would move the tarantata to express her crisis.

Luigi Stifani explained how he had once played for a tarantata for hours and hours without being able to elicit any kind of response. Eventually, following a hunch, he struck up Chopin's funeral march and, to his own and everyone else's surprise, the afflicted jumped up and danced. 'When she recovered,' Stifani concluded with an indignant smile, 'she asked me why I hadn't played Chopin's piece straight away!'[20] In some cases, rhythmic stimulation, not intended as music, was sufficient to bring about a response and, with it, a resurgence of symptoms: footsteps on the floor of a tobacco factory incited one tarantata to dance; a spoon hitting the sides of a bowl provoked another (De Martino 2005: 56, 58). Many, I was repeatedly told, avoided social occasions at which the pizzica was played during periods in which they felt particularly sensitive, and hence at risk of falling into a crisis outside a contained ritual framework.

Music helped identify the cause of affliction. 'You no longer saw a man, but a scorpion instead. It brought tears to our eyes to see him like this.' Luigi Stifani relates his experience of playing for a tarantato bitten by a scorpion.[21] The tarantate were said to become their predator: mostly a spider, sometimes other poisonous animals. Where everyday roles faltered, the spider and its counterparts provided role models catering to extremes of behaviour. In fact, diverse tarantula types existed in the context of tarantism rituals, providing scope for individual and historical variation. Each spider carried its own name and traits, determining the conduct of its victims. Dancing and singing tarantulas were most common. Others were angry or promiscuous, pushing the tarantate to aggressive or lustful behaviour. Yet others were sad and silent, responding only to funeral laments. Some were sleepy and even deaf, showing no reaction to music at all (Mina 1997). A varied costume cupboard of characters existed, determining the behaviour, wishes and whims of the tarantula's prey.

But what was it about the music that made it 'right'? For centuries this question has intrigued researchers interested in the link between music and healing (Kircher 1641/1654; Katner 1952; Rouget 1986; Franco and Zuffi 1996). Was it the type of instrument or rhythm used, the melodic range or musical mode? Some musicians informed De Martino (2005: 299) that the tonality of the music played was crucial. The tarantate apparently responded mainly to musical pieces in specific keys: A major, D major, B minor and A minor. De Martino himself did not observe this, and I am equally unable to provide any confirmation. It seems clear that some highly subjective associations, as well as cultural conventions come into play, as, 'by itself, music cannot alter the consciousness of those who are neither sensitized to it nor expectant of its results' (Laderman 1996: 132).

However, a general preference for fast rhythms established the pizzica as a favourite. Luigi Stifani (2000: 39) spoke of three types he used most in his career: *la tarantata indiavolata* and *la tarantata sorda*, the 'possessed or devilish' and 'deaf' forms, played in a major key; and *la tarantata minore*, performed in a minor key. The basic beat of the pizzica was also said to hold clues to ritual efficacy. Despite its 4/4 rhythm, varying accents give it a 6/8 feel, making its structure dual and ambiguous: four counts per bar overlaid with uneven triplets create a jumpy feel, characteristic of the skipping steps for which the tarantella dance is famous. The name pizzica pizzica itself gives a sense, moreover, of the triple rhythm of this music and dance form. Generally speaking, a continuous rhythm, diversely accentuated, came with melodic variants, improvisational in character. The instruments reflected this duality: the musical beat, set by the tambourine, was accompanied by an interweaving offbeat, generally provided by the violin. Accordions, harmonicas or guitars contributed further sound variety, although already a reduced selection from bygone centuries, in which musettes, shawms, trumpets, bombardons and other wind instruments were equally part of the game (De Martino 2005: 97).[22]

Importantly, moreover, not all music was instrumental. Singing tarantate required vocals: declarations of love, funeral laments, religious hymns, and, most of all, evocations of the tarantula or St Paul through prayers or verbal dialogues, expressed aloud or silently. What is more, definitions of musical props were put to the test by the soundscape inside St Paul's chapel. Musical instruments were officially forbidden, but personal accounts contradict this (Di Lecce 1994: 242). The apostle's brides became their own musicians. Their screams and sighs mixed with the singing of songs and the clapping of hands. Recurring cries of just two syllables, 'A-hi', punctuated their efforts at ritualization.[23] Images transported in the words of songs were said to provide other steps towards identification and recovery.[24]

Yet other props helped to re-evoke the tarantula, including the reconstruction of the setting and scene of the first bite. Objects present and clothes worn at the moment of the initial crisis became crucial props, as did icons of St Paul, mirrors, leaves, twigs or water. Swinburne (1783) adds ribbons and grapes to this list. Fragrances provided yet other tools: a young man believed to be a tarantato was seen to place a bunch of wild flowers close to his nose as if 'trying to obtain a stimulation through smell which did not come through hearing or sight' (De Martino 2005: 50). Another tarantata reported how, under the tarantula's spell, she became intolerant to certain smells (ibid.: 58).

Chromatic explorations provided further clues, as the case of the man ejected during Maria of Nardò's ritual recalls. Coloured props acted as both magnets and repellents, determining the colour of the afflicting spider. Most important for this were coloured ribbons, *nzacareddhe* in the Salentine dialect. These are still sold as signs of devotion at religious festivals. De Martino (2005: 106) writes of diversely coloured bits of material suspended from a string tied across the ritual perimeter. The tarantate chose those that most affected them. According to Kircher's text (1641/1654), some ravaged pieces of cloth with their teeth or embraced them lovingly.

Moreover, every move was made in the tarantula's name. A conceptual jump was taken to establish dramatic or ritual distance. The tarantata both was and was not herself. Choreographic ritual cycles, initiated by musical rhythms and the tarantate's identificatory actions, generally began with a slow section and then broke into a faster rhythm. In the first phase, performed on the ground, widespread interpretations suggest that the spirit of the tarantula, or offending counterpart, was called upon and brought alive through the process of embodiment. The spider was made visual and tangible through identification with its shape and movements: the tarantula-tarantata would arch her spine into a 'hysteric arc', shuffle across the floor on her back and shoulders with her limbs stretched out spiderlike, dance with a cushion above her shoulder, apparently representing the arachnid torso, or swing suspended from a rope. Alternatively, she was known for the feat of threading her entire body through the legs of a wicker chair, in simulation of the spider's weaving skills.

Other movements characterizing rituals were seen to foster identification, as well as a sense of disorientation and a loss of balance, common to dance forms found in other regions of the world associated with so-called altered states of consciousness, often compared to the spider's dance (De Martino 1961a; Lewis 1971; Bourguignon 1973; Rouget 1986; Lapassade 1994, 1996a; Ardillo 1997; Daniel 2005). These included throwing the head from side to side; moving the pelvis rapidly up and down; running or dancing in a circle; or spinning around in a pirouette.[25]

In a second dance phase performed in an upright position, the spider dancer was said to enter into battle, as some interpretations relate. She had to face her predator, fight and eliminate it. Dance steps of the pizzica pizzica were seen to trample and crush the spider, as the heel hit the ground rapidly and forcefully, until the dancer collapsed from exhaustion and rested before recommencing another cycle. The performance ended when the spider was pacified. A complete and permanent cure, popular opinion states, was obtained only when the spider was killed.

In more recent centuries, the role of the spider has merged with that of the Apostle Paul, a further protagonist in the tarantula's dance. Luigi Chiriatti writes of how some, drawing on this association, were known to say prayers to St Paul whenever they came across a spider web (1995: 56). The apostle is frequently described as *lo sposo delle tarantate*, the spouse of the tarantate, providing one explanation for the white dress, the colour of a bride's gown in recent centuries, identifying his female devotees. Their costume and money offerings became dramatic media to seduce the saint at Galatina, as moments of identification and antagonism continued to emerge. Allusions to sexual intercourse, especially during the initial dance phase on the floor, as well as the erotic connotations of some lyrics, evoked St Paul's presence, as did other dramatic techniques: many approached the altar on their knees; one tarantata was filmed pounding on the door behind which St Paul's statue stood; others climbed onto the altar to be closer to the tapestry that bore his image. In the second phase, the saint was challenged: one tarantata was captured on celluloid as she circled the altar in Galatina's chapel, whipping a white handkerchief through the air as if to chase away her aggressor [see Fig. 1.3], while others used moves of the *scherma* to fight invisible counterparts (Chiriatti 1996: 12; De Martino 2005: 103).

Props and techniques provided key clues to ritual efficacy, but so did the active participation of others. De Martino (2005: 104) presents the musical performers as exorcists, medics and artists all in one, mentioning how – apparently – 'in seventeenth-century Taranto, the musicians were public officials paid with regular salaries' (2005: 183). More commonly, musicians were remunerated and fed by the victim's family, causing major expenses. In the past, both men and women played for the tarantate, and rituals relied on their dexterity: not only their technical skills but also their ability to instil the performance with an emotional charge and to let go of any compulsion to control in order to submit to the needs of the tarantata involved. At some point, one elderly musician reported, the musicians themselves were taken over by the music. Something else played through them.[26]

Vital knowledge about how to safeguard the ritual sequence was often provided by close family members or others who had extensive ritual experience. Luigi Santoro (1982: 81) points to the centrality of the figure of the *macara*, while Turchini (1987: 162) refers to the *capo-attarantati*, the head of the attarantati, who ensured that appropriate action was taken and organized ritual practicalities. Friends and relatives also took on responsibility for the safety and well-being of the afflicted: catching the tarantate when they collapsed, supplying food and drink, securing the scene from potential intruders and paying the musicians' fees. Moreover, bystanders or other tarantate could be invited to join in the dance. In fact, historical documents tell of large groups of afflicted dancers dressing up and dancing in crowds (Baldwin 1997).

Representatives of larger institutions have been equally influential within the complex play of tarantism, often restricting performative efficacy. Priests were encouraged to dissuade the tarantate from coming to Galatina, although others were invited to perform exorcism rituals. De Martino mentions how one tarantato was stopped in mid-dance because the collection of money during rituals was no longer authorized (2005: 53). During St Paul's festival the police curbed proceedings, calling the tarantate to order, keeping crowds at bay, or placating relatives enraged by journalists and photographers.

Following the publication of *La terra del rimorso*, journalists and researchers arrived with their props of cameras, tape recorders and microphones. Their dramatic techniques often implied trickery, as some hid on the balcony inside St Paul's chapel to film from behind a concealing curtain or smuggled themselves inside the chapel on the pretence of being relatives or musicians. Gianfranco Mingozzi's film *Sulla terra del rimorso* (1982) documents how a film team lured the reluctant and infuriated Maria of Nardò into her doctor's practice to interview her, while the narrator justifies this as legitimate for the sake of documenting 'the existence of a subaltern class which in many cases has not as yet acquired a sense of self-consciousness, and is unable to provide a direct testimony of itself without external mediators' (Barbati et al. 1978: 142).[27] Such patronizing views justified invasive techniques. These may explain the antagonism towards film cameras expressed by the tarantate, beyond questions about the extent to which this antagonism may have been triggered by class issues, in so far as those using the cameras may have represented a particular level of technological development and the inadvertent display of the financial means to acquire such technology.[28]

In sum, ritual efficacy in bygone ritual contexts required both physical and conceptual containment. Although the afflicted essentially directed proceedings through their reactions, everyone present played an active role as a witness: as potential critic or accomplice. No matter what motive pulled them into the circle – be it curiosity, reverence or condemnation – any act of observing reconfirmed what was happening. As long as those present were willing to acknowledge the performative reality of the ritual setting, or at least refrained from denying it, they played a crucial role in promoting ritual efficacy and safeguarding the acceptability of this tradition. Where in past rituals the right thread had to be found, the 'right air' needs to be struck in contemporary performances: that way and intensity of playing which binds the audience's attention and compels participants to dance and applaud.

175

Showbiz Airs: Present Props and Techniques

With the 1990s' pizzica boom, the new or neo-tarantati emerged. 'All are looking for a state of grace,' Daniele Durante (1999: 172) writes, 'almost of trance, which can put them in relation with their own divinity, or demon, or the tarantula or St Rocco.' This is not the only motivation, but one that highlights the persisting star position of symbolic and spiritual counterparts. Images of these counterparts abound and the tarantula still holds prime position, unchallenged at the 'top of the pops', on tambourine skins, billboards, posters, ashtrays or book and CD covers. In 2002, a bar on Galatina's main square displayed sweets shaped as spiders, calendars of the tarantate and T-shirts with their perpetrators. A market vendor with a spider sticker on his chest pocket sold others, at one euro each, among his selection of nuts and olives.

Meanwhile, the newsagent across the road had a large selection of postcards with tambourines, some smeared with blood, and verses of songs addressing St Paul and the tarantula, while the spider advertising the 2007 Night of the Tarantula on billboards throughout the region also sold at 30 euros as a silver pendant in an elegant jewellery shop in Lecce's old city centre. The tarantula remains a buzzword, a magnet, a label. It has become history and memory inscribed on human skin: Pino Zimba, recently deceased leader of the group Zimbaria, had a spider tattooed onto his shoulder at the point where his father was bitten.[29] Sometimes actual spiders have become inadvertent actors in a show, as one musician told how he had caught a tarantula and taken it to every performance of his band.[30]

Saints, such as Paul or Rocco, maintain a more marginal role. Some nuovi tarantati visit St Paul's Galatina chapel on his feast day and hundreds make their annual pilgrimage to St Rocco's festival without, however, necessarily entering the chapel safeguarding the saint's relics. The documentary film *San Paolo e la tarantola* concludes with the final acknowledgement: 'Mit besonderem Dank an San Paolo' (With special thanks to St Paul), as director Edoardo Winspeare, then a film-school student in Munich, resurrected the tarantate's patron on cinema and television screens.

Meanwhile, the 'dancing shaman' of the Porto Badisco caves is another favourite embellishment [see Figs 7.1 and 7.2]. In the eyes of some, the longevity of this cave painting outweighs that of the spider, symbolically making it a predecessor, a kind of source, with an archaeological halo of mystery augmenting its charisma. In the 1998 summer, a bright-red graffiti design of this figure stood out on the walls of a small, makeshift bar erected next to the largest inlet of Badisco, just a few strides from the iron-barred cave entrance [see Fig. 7.1]. The following year, this bar was turned into a regular brick building at the expense of the shaman, as his image was torn down with the initial walls. However, his graffiti-style presence is alive and kicking in the Salentine music scene. 'This figure,' Daniele Durante (1999: 189) explains, 'has struck the imagination of the Salentine people to such an extent, as to identify it with the divinity which they consider to be at the origin of their ... culture ... it is in the pizzica that they see its "still-beating heart".' While many Salentines would not grant the shaman such a monopoly, such historical associations provide perfect tools for grounding today's performances in the past and in the territory of the Salento itself.

Although the ancient Greek roots of tarantism are widely defended by academics (Salvatore 1989; Lapassade 1994; Di Mitri 1996), few, if any, images relating to the Greek world are visible within the contemporary manifestations of tarantism, although the lyrics of many songs in the *Griko* dialect – and Greek radio channels picked up across the Otranto channel when driving along the Adriatic coast – are a constant reminder of the Salento's (cultural) proximity to Greek shores.

The tambourine remains a key prop loaded with free-floating meanings not necessarily shared and not necessarily rooted in everyday life. Students participating at the 1998 University of Lecce pizzica course directed by Giorgio Di Lecce spoke of these associations: 'It's an expression of energy inside ... an extension of our own voice ... something that carries you away.'[31] 'I check my pulse prior to starting to play the tambourine,' another musician asserts, suggesting an intrinsic link between the tambourine's rhythm and human heartbeat.[32] Fabio Tolledi (1998: 4) takes up this thread: 'The tambourine, symbolic form of the cosmos, holds in its beat the relation that exists between the heart and the world.' 'The secret is the tambourine,' yet another player affirms:

> It is round, like the moon. It is a feminine instrument. Its skin is generally made from the stomach of an animal, the stomach being at the centre of all

living things, where the emotions are, where children are formed. The hand is used to play on this skin. Stretched out open wide, it has the shape of a spider. The spider beats the tambourine, in the centre, in the stomach, giving it a strong, continuous rhythm, following the beat of the heart.'[33]

Such associations connect instruments, spiders and players, jeopardizing frequently expressed exclusive links between the pizzica and those born and bred in the Salento.[34]

Part of the tambourine's secret is believed to lie in the experiences it is seen to provoke. Hands are generally bound with protective strips of cloth, but these may loosen and the skin below the thumb is frequently cut open from the friction of beating the instrument. Many players tell how they continued playing with a bleeding hand because they felt no pain and, in fact, many tambourine skins are smeared with dried blood. Voices express marvel at the fact that pain is annulled and this too is charged with broader meanings, as Tolledi (1998: 8) reveals:

> There exists among tambourine players a cruel and childish kind of pride with regard to the 'baptism' of those who play this instrument. This sonic virginity is broken by admission into the sphere of adult players by the blood which bleeds from the hand, and by the red … which colours and signs the tambourine. The hand becomes a sign, many signs, a wound which opens and bleeds, a red mouth, an open sex.

From this perspective, bleeding becomes an initiation and rite of passage facilitated by playing the tambourine and a means of inscribing a change from youth to adult status. Associations are made with women's loss of virginity, a highly charged bodily metaphor for the vulnerability of social boundaries. Yet one might wonder whether past performers went to such extremes when hard manual labour was awaiting them the next day and their hands were, moreover, much more resistant from work.

Meanwhile, the human voice too remains a central device, as Daniele Durante (1999: 175) stresses:

> Used as an instrument with tightly stretched chords … verses lose their original significance; they are extrapolated from other songs and interspersed with cries, exclamations, which at times seem animalesque verses. Often 'mamma' is added to the 'A-hi' to obtain 'A-hi mamma!', an ancestral exclamation which, each time it is pronounced, produces an inexplicable excitement in the players with a subsequent increase in the sound volume.

Lyrics are also highly significant. One dancer explained how these vary between the pizzica pizzica and scherma: 'When the pizzica is danced for courtship, lyrics speak of love, encouraging dancers to give of their best, but, when it is performed for the scherma, words are much more aggressive, aiming to inspire anger, tension and courage.'[35]

Inevitably, money is also a prime prop, often determining whether a performance will be staged at all. In 2006, one of the key groups of the tarantula's music and dance was asking between 1,000 euros and 2,600 euros for one night's concert, depending on whether they were playing locally or elsewhere, with events outside the Salento generally being a better bet financially. One well-known and charismatic elderly musician, is said to ask up to 2,500 euros for a single appearance, even when playing in the Salento. Specific events may be bigger scoops, such as playing during election campaigns, for EU-funded projects or on the Night of the Tarantula, while other occasions may involve voluntary participation, often linked to an exchange of favours. For most, playing is a sideline income, considering that these sums are shared among group members and may or may not include travel expenses. Many groups have brought out their own CDs, involving average expenditures of 300 euros per day for the use of a recording studio, not to speak of the time invested by group members, although sales subsequently contribute to concert incomes and publicity. Yet others have specialized in book and music sales concerning the tarantula and spend the summer months touring concert venues.

City and regional sponsorship have made certain events highly attractive for participants: in 2002, the first Salentine edition of Estadanza, a rich one-week programme of practical and theoretical courses on the tarantula's music and dance, directed by dance ethnologist Giuseppe Gala in collaboration with various local associations, cost no more than 100 euros including accommodation, with further discounts available for those resident in the Salento. Meanwhile for participants, concerts are generally free in the Salento, whereas abroad entrance fees are frequently charged: London's Rhythm and Sticks Festival sold £15 (22 euros) tickets for the performance of Salentine group Ghetonia on 20 July 2004. Meanwhile, the audience at the Beijing Night of the Tarantula on 2 May 2006 paid 30 yuan (almost 3 euros) each (Indennitate 2006).

The Provincia di Lecce's expenditure of 100,000 euros for this latter event inevitably created polemical reactions, with a spokesman for the Lecce town council provocatively offering a piazza in Lecce at only 20,000 euros for the same concert (Meis 2006).

The role of technological advances is equally important to the success of contemporary performances. 'Not only must acoustics be good for the audience,' one musician stresses, 'but it is just as important that performers hear themselves and each other.'[36] In this sense, today's groups are often in the hands of more or less skilled sound technicians and their show is influenced by other factors such as the amplification system available or sound pollution from elsewhere. At the same time, technology amplifies communicative means. The group Alla Bua was one of the first to play to the backdrop of their music video, while the Night of the Tarantula has involved huge screens duplicating and zooming in on what was happening on stage, while the entire concert was broadcast worldwide on satellite TV. Internet sites and forums provide other virtual performance spaces and avenues for venting opinions, creating contacts, exchanging information.

Moreover, the importance of the immediacy and flexibility of the musical source is spotlighted. The interaction or mutual 'reactivity' that is possible between live players and dancers, and was transmitted from older to younger generations in the past, is less direct when a mechanical source of music is used. 'A good performance', another musician points out, 'depends not only on the sound being good both on and off stage, but also on a circuit of attention and enthusiasm between audience and musicians.'[37] Although technological devices may record and fix musical pieces on discs and digital files, and many DJs master the technical possibilities of interacting with their crowds of fans, they cannot make up for a live performance's creative and improvisatory emotional charge and rhythm.[38]

A tambourine maker and maestro player from Ostuni expands on this point:

> The other day, a music group from further south came to give a concert here in my hometown, but nobody was dancing. The group leader shouted to me to come and play with them. We began to play the pizzica of our town, slowly, gently, not in an unrestrained way ... The pizzica is life, it has its own rhythms and if you don't speak the same language you must find the way, the air, the intonation to speak. You might have the instrument and everything else, but the right air is missing, the right motive.[39]

The 'right air' has to be found, that rhythm and intention, that way of playing which will engage those present to take part, beginning with the tapping of toes on the piazza pavement or the barely visible swaying of shoulders.

> The right air must be adapted not only to the individual and group but also to the place where music making takes place. Someone may enter a circle limping and then begin to take in the air, to gain confidence, to let go and to show themselves in all their grandeur. But, if the right air is lost, the pizzica no longer makes anyone dance.[40]

With the contemporary pizzica boom, 'official' (and often disputed) pizzica courses abound, but these aspects of performing may not always be addressed. Many become involved in the pizzica world, moreover, without ever seeking out a tutor: 'A typical introductory route is through friends: you take part for the first time, you get carried away by the music and dance, you continue to dance and begin to read books without giving it too much thought. Then you learn to play the tambourine and so on.'[41] In either case, there are no guidelines or guarantee that implicit rules alluded to by the elderly are acquired. Another musician elaborates further on the transmission of the pizzica:

> The dimension of experience, trance for instance, is an individual thing, which is then transmitted. We exchange experiences. We talk about them afterwards. Trance takes you into superior situations, it puts you into contact with another world, with another universe, it's a magical fact and therefore a bit difficult to explain scientifically, technically. But, for us who have lived these things, it's almost a natural fact. However, to arrive at this point, it's necessary to respect certain rules: the contact with the earth, the natural terrain, the circle, players who are all keeping to the same rhythms. Also, a minimum of two hours of playing is needed before accessing any state of trance. Then you arrive at this energy, which rotates, which engages first one person and then another.[42]

Sufficient stamina, perfect rhythm and lengthy playing are said to be required. 'It's not only a matter of studying the tambourine, of learning about harmony,' the same musician continues. 'It's a matter of understanding what happens around you. These things the old people transmitted to you, both by speaking and by placing themselves next to you, by playing beside you'.[43] The importance of creating an emotional charge is emphasized, as is the need to

181

maintain a 'sonorous flow'. In line with this, Luigi Toma explains that nowadays his group rarely inserts a break during concerts: 'If I stop playing, I find it very difficult to start up again. It becomes an enormous effort, because this state in which the rhythm takes over ceases and then you have to work hard to return to it again. That's why I almost always forego a break.'[44]

Clearly, ways of performing vary widely, influencing what may be defined as a successful performance. Such success, in turn, depends on the criteria applied and who defines these. Inevitably, gender issues are brought into play too. Once a fellow female dancer corrected one of my dance steps, specifying that it was a man's step: 'The pizzica is danced in an unchained but never in an unseemly way. It mustn't become vulgar. You don't show your legs. There must always be elegance and composure.'[45] Not only do gender differences appear but also generational ones, as Ada's description of her eighty-four-year-old mother's way of dancing shows [see Fig. 5.1]:

> She moves proudly, and at the same time with great humility towards her male partner. It is a way of dancing the pizzica that is entirely female. We, the new generation, have learned that we also have a masculine side and how to express this. Elderly women, however, will never take on masculine modes, as we do. They have a proud comportment, making sure to keep their legs very closed, taking tiny but very sensual steps. This was the role of women at the time, and they could not move beyond it.[46]

Changes inevitably jeopardize implicit rules once associated with the pizzica, and attempts at reinforcing these are often in vain, as Ada recounts:

> I tried ... but realized that nothing could be done. It's not possible to say: 'Look, it's not done like that, it's done like this,' because in that moment they'll tell you: 'I want to dance, move out of my way, I have to dance and I want to enter the circle.' In this way, twenty, thirty people dance in one circle and there is too much energy, it's not channelled in any way, it's chaos.'[47]

Tradition dictates that only one couple dance in a circle at one time. They become the nucleus of attention, holding each other's gaze and dancing without ever touching beyond slight brushes of the skin. Stimuli – whistles, applause, cries of admiration, laughter and more – are directed at the dancing couple from the audience, creating constant interaction. Yet, inevitably, the open and improvisatory character of the pizzica steps and gestures easily overrides any disciplinary structures at its base, leading Giuseppe Gala (2002b: 46) to cynically describe the pizzica (or *pizziche*) today, as involving 'a television-like emphasis on representing the relationship of couples: the exaggeratingly honeyed female role and the sugary gaze of men who drone around their prey'.

Clearly, no essentialized pizzica exists. Intentions vary, as do ways of performing. Obvious performative similarities between past and present spider dances, based on sounds, steps and lyrics, are permeated with deeply rooted differences, which go beyond the dynamic and continuously re-creative character that applies to any performance genre. Modern technology provides a vast new gamut of virtual, rather than live, stimuli. Moreover, the human organism, the key prop of the tarantula's music and dance, is exposed not only to highly varied individual experiences, but also to disparate sociocultural contexts. Contemporary performers not only may lack stamina, but also play in a context that lends the tarantula's music and dance to whatever interpretation is at hand, making a ballet-school ritual copy the highlight of a night. Knowing about roots and rhythms cannot replace the experiential knowledge of appropriate relations assuring containment that the elderly talk about.

Ritual set-ups guaranteed a minimum of support: perimeters were clearly demarcated, musicians played in a circle, someone experienced guided and secured the proceedings, throwing out intruders if need be. Today, performance circles are often crowded with participants ignorant of the value of someone directing interactions. Stages and amplifying systems split participants, and attempts at bridging gaps with performers descending into the crowd or inviting audience members on stage may only underline and deepen divisions. The tarantula's music not only welds together but also breaks apart, as the strong rivalry among contemporary music groups repeatedly brings to the fore. Luigi Toma refers to this emphatically: 'Why is it that all of us who live in the Salento don't manage to work together? This is the basis of our music! At this point, we're all taking ourselves for a ride!'[48]

The comparative perspective adopted here may be criticized as perpetuating wishful thinking regarding the continuity of those performative features perceived as beneficial by whoever is promoting these events. Although similarities emerge, these are no guarantee of historical or cultural ties between bygone and modern tarantati. What was right in the past is not necessarily right nowadays. What is appropriate for one person is not necessarily so for another. What is interesting, however, is how a focus on continuity – and a demand for this – can both obscure and reveal the inherent power of performances: that is, the creative potential, or possibility for discontinuity and change, implicit in every new enactment.

Inevitably, criteria of success depend on who establishes these. Nevertheless, it appears that performative efficacy – despite variations in past and present contexts and in participants (whether Salentine or not) – is linked to a sensitivity towards places, times, props and techniques gained through extensive experiential knowledge. It is facilitated by the active participation of everyone present; the anchoring of performances in social and natural rhythms of everyday life; and the availability of performance techniques related to the larger socio-natural context as well as containment, sensory stimulation and emotional charge. A key to success emerges in the way of playing and the intention behind doing so.

The importance of surrendering to the music in the circles of musicians and dancers, moreover, comes into view, juxtaposed to the management of music and dance through cultural politics and policies, as well as artistic directives and arrangements: relinquishing control as opposed to controlling; abandonment versus regulation; letting go in the face of legislation; a paradox engulfed by the tarantula's web and, perhaps, an opposition inherent in the process of recovering well-being.[49]

Notes

1. See Schieffelin (1996) for a discussion of 'failure' and 'efficiency' in performance. The notion of technique, meanwhile, may be divided into two overlapping categories, mutually shaping each other: daily techniques, habitual ways of acting appropriated through socialization (Mauss 1979), and extra-daily techniques acquired through performance training, which 'literally *put* the body *into form*, rendering it artificial/artistic but *believable*' (Barba 1995: 16).
2. Nardò, 29 July 1999.
3. The meaning of this sign remains ambivalent in Italian: it may be translated as both 'cultural study on tarantism' or 'workshop for the study of tarantism culture.'
4. Other sites dedicated to the Apostle Paul include the towns of Acaya and Alessano (Torsello 1997a; Nocera 2005).
5. In March 2005, the chapel of St Paul was selected by Il Fondo Ambiente Italia, the Italian Environmental Fund, as a key site to be safeguarded from ruin. Thanks to the initiative of the Centro Studi sul Tarantismo in Galatina, the chapel of St Paul was elected in seventeenth position on a national scale of *Luoghi del cuore*, Places of the heart, a campaign inviting citizens to nominate places of particular beauty worthy of preservation but at risk of being forgotten, in a nationwide census (Trono 2005).
6. For reprints of these documents, see Lüdtke (2000b).
7. Alessano, 10 August 2005. The speaker uses the Italian phrase *una sensibilità dei luoghi*.
8. Tricase, 20 May 1998.
9. Casarano, 29 May 1998.
10. Tricase, 20 May 1998.
11. Ibid.
12. Personal communication.
13. Ostuni, 10 July 1999.
14. Depressa, 4 May 1998.
15. Ostuni, 10 July 1999.
16. See Chapter 4, 'La Sagra dei Curli: a Community Festival'.
17. Galatina, 28 June 1999.
18. 11 August 1999.
19. The Pizzicata Festival was staged from 1999 to 2003, with the final concert initially located in the idyllic surroundings of the rural church of Santa Marina di Stigliano, near Carpignano Salentino. In 2000, it involved a trans-European programme funded by the EU Leader II Programme, including workshops with musicians and dancers from Ireland and Brittany. This event was seen by some as a counter-initiative to the Night of the Tarantula.

20. Nardò, 29 July 1999.
21. Ibid.
22. It is important to keep in mind that 'the terms for instruments have undergone numerous changes through the centuries, and the same term in one period could also refer to very different instruments in different geographical areas' (Dorothy Zinn in De Martino 2005: 92).
23. A short record was sold with De Martino's first edition of *La terra del rimorso* (1961a), documenting sounds registered in St Paul's chapel on 29 June 1959 and several musical pieces and songs performed during rituals. Likewise, Brizio Montinaro's collection *Musiche e canti popolari del Salento*, Vol. 3 (Edizioni Aramirè), includes two tracks of recordings (from 1974 and earlier) of the tarantate in Galatina.
24. De Martino distinguished three such steps towards recovery in one of the tarantate's famous hymns 'Santu Paulu meu de le tarante': first, the evocation of the presence of the causative agent: 'Say where the tarantula stung you'; secondly, the localization of the embodied crisis: 'Underneath the hem of the skirt'; and, finally, the presentation of a resolution by calling upon St Paul, 'who stings all the girls and makes them saints' (De Martino 2005: 99–100).
25. Maurizio Nocera, Lecce, 24 November 1997.
26. Nardò, 6 July 1999.
27. The dialogue, narrated text and a description of this film's image sequences are found in Barbati et al. (1978: 115–44).
28. I thank Marina Roseman for bringing this point to my attention.
29. Aradeo, 10 September 1998.
30. Muro Leccese, 10 September 1998.
31. Lecce, 12 March 1998.
32. Cisternino, 3 May 1998.
33. Galatina, 29 June 1999.
34. Such connections between musical and cardiac rhythms are similarly drawn elsewhere: Marina Roseman (2002: 119) stresses the central role of bamboo-tube stampers in Temiar trance dances and how the rhythms of these instruments are compared to the rhythms of heartbeat and breathing.
35. Casamasella, 16 August 1998. See, for example, the first two verses of the song 'Sta cala lu serenu':
    'Sta cala lu serenu de le stelle, e quista è la notte ca rrubba le donne. Ci rrubba donne nu se chiama ladru, se chiama giovanottu 'nnamurato. Intra sta curte nc'è na fina perla. Passu la riveriscu e nu me parla. Se 'ncete qualche amante la pretenda. Dinni cu se rigira a l'autra vanda. Ca ieu me lu cumbattu cu la scherma. Percè me l'ha prumisa la soa mamma.'
    (Evening mists are falling from the stars, this is the night to conquer women. Whoever conquers women isn't called a thief; he's called a young man in

love ... In this courtyard there is a fine pearl. I pass to see her but she doesn't speak to me. If she has a lover who wants her, tell him to go around the other way. I will fight him with the scherma, because her mother has promised her to me.)

36. Lecce, 19 October 2005.
37. Ibid.
38. A parallel can be drawn here to Katherine Hagedorn's (2001) study of Cuban Santería stressing how 'spontaneity and improvisation, fundamental components of sacred musical practice, often tend to be lost in the move to regulate culture for consumption by a broader public' (Moore 2003: 154).
39. Ostuni, 10 July 1999.
40. Ibid.
41. Galatina, 29 June 1999.
42. Tricase, 20 May 1998.
43. Ibid.
44. Casarano, 29 May 1998.
45. Galatina, 29 June 1999.
46. Torrepaduli, 19 August 1999.
47. Ibid.
48. Casarano, 29 May 1998.
49. Drama therapist Sue Jennings (1995: 188) confirms: 'It is the capacity of the therapist/shaman/actor to allow "controlled abandon" that enables healing potential within the therapeutic space.'

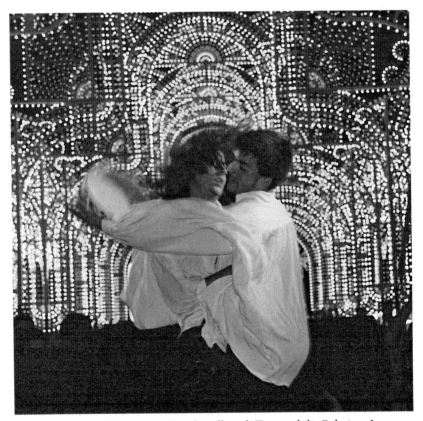

Fig. 8.1 Concert of the group I Tamburellisti di Torrepaduli, Galatina, June 1999 (photo: Karen Lüdtke).

Chapter 8
SpiderWoMen Transformed: Celebrating Well-being

> When you let go of your hand, the tambourine starts playing;
> when you let go of your voice, the song starts singing;
> and when you let go of your body, the pizzica starts dancing.
>
> Giorgio Di Lecce, Lecce, 12 March 1998

In July 2004 the Rhythm and Sticks Festival, celebrating percussion music from around the world, brought the pizzica to the South Bank Centre, one of London's major arts and culture venues. The well-known Salentine group Ghetonia made its debut in the UK capital, performing its repertoire of songs in the *Griko* dialect and pieces featuring the rhythmic beat of the pizzica. The Purcell Room auditorium with its black-curtained walls contrasted sharply with the open-air settings of the Salento, but the concert was a huge success. The musicians interacted humorously with the audience and their pieces were enthusiastically received, with a standing ovation at the end. What really stood out for me, however, was a split-second interaction right at the end of the performance: as the musicians got back on stage for an encore and were about to strike their instruments, a member of the audience jumped to his feet, in a jack-in-the-box fashion, brandishing between his outstretched arms a bright red and yellow scarf – the colours of the Lecce football team – which read: 'Forza Lecce!' (Come on, Lecce!).

Beyond its comic effect, this gesture pinpointed a Salentine émigré's strong sense of (or desire for) belonging, with his football paraphrenalia, and, by way of association, may be seen to have rooted this music and all it entails within the Salento. All the more potent in the cosmopolitan setting of London's South Bank Centre and in the context of an international 'world music' festival, this gesture could be viewed as creating and shaping not only geographical boundaries, but also symbolic and imaginary territories, zones of inclusion and exclusion, bringing to the fore questions of identity and the perceived need for identity within the modern-day world. In order to consider how identities are played out in relation to well-being in the contexts of the tarantula's music and dance, it is useful to gradually zoom outwards from individual experiences, to social relations and, finally, group identities. Such a widening of the focal lens reveals the mutual influence between these various dynamic and entwined dimensions.

As the sensory modalities of touch, sound, colour, motion and smell are engaged, participants in the pizzica's rhythms may move from one experiential state to another. Affliction may shape-shift to well-being, addressing not only individual suffering but also 'scars of history' (Roseman 1996: 234) on a communal level. In this sense, the tarantula's music and dance reveal themselves as one example of how, in the context of modernity, both in the Salento and elsewhere, 'people are mediating the simultaneous yet differentiated, overlapped, and overlaid world of transnational communication and global economies' (Roseman 2002: 121). Performance circles seen to evoke a sense of 'magic' are fundamental in this process.

Magic Circles: Allowing Music to Take Over

A focus on magic circles, or *ronde magiche*, allows us to zoom in on individual experiences seen to promote well-being.[1] Such magic circles may emerge on any occasion in which the tarantula's music and dance are performed.[2] Generally speaking, however, big-time on-stage shows appear less conducive to such magic emerging, due to their highly structured nature, although even in these contexts participants both on and off stage may allude to such experiences.

Two young female dancers relate what they have lived:

The experience of participating in these circles becomes something mystical and fascinating. The circle creates a harmony of sounds, bodies, emotions ... everybody gives and takes energy in a quasi-symbiotic exchange with the others and with the music. For those who dance, this pursuit also becomes spatial and the arms, legs, head, every tiniest part of the body, amplify their receptivity. (Negro and Sergio 2000: 1)

'It's a question of knowing how to create a circle, *una ronda*,' stresses one Salentine musician, 'a question of going beyond tiredness. Then you enter into a different dimension, a dimension of spirituality.'[3]

These views underline the fact that active participation and personal experience – based on the gradual acquisition not only of technical abilities, but also of experiential knowledge and implicitly embodied rules – provide a key to gaining an ability of feeling and finding the 'right air'. Another musician explains: 'It's impossible to say what exactly brings out this magic. It's unpredictable. You just have to be ready, without expecting anything.'[4] Luigi Toma adds:

> There has to be a real sense of explosion. Anybody can have a beautiful voice and sing. Anybody can know how to play the tambourine, but the emotional charge may not be there, this interior charge which is transmitted. You feel the impact physically, directly. You have to let yourself go when you play, without thinking about the people that are watching you.'[5]

Daniele Durante (1999: 173–74) expands on this in his account of playing in contemporary contexts, making a clear distinction between on-stage concert settings and performance circles in which the musician (more often than not a man) is immersed in the crowd of dancers and spectators: 'He mustn't make himself noticeable, he must "function" and that's it! He must create a flow, which isn't ever interrupted, into which the dancers can enter, feeling themselves carried away to perform gestures and movements without worrying about who might look at or judge them.' The musicians must place themselves at the service of the music and the dancers – reminiscent of ritual players who spoke of 'music taking over'.

Such 'circles of musicians, singers and dancers', Daniele Durante (1999: 168–72) continues:

> are attributed a magical valence, which assured a cure from any kind of illness to all active participants … What matters is not the technical ability of the musician or the grace of a single dancer, but the total effect … that of a cyclical music … of an incessant rhythm … instilling a magical process with which it is possible to enchant and imprison certain forces and to exorcize others.

So-called magical dynamics may be invisible to the eye, but are nevertheless experienced as highly tangible and real by participants.

In the past, these dynamics were ascribed to the tarantula or St Paul, as their victims appeared to be at the mercy of the tunes preferred by their particular aggressor. Stephen Storace (1753) told how he unexpectedly found himself playing his violin for a tarantata despite his ignorance of the tunes required. As someone else sang, he tried out the notes on his instrument and immediately impelled the afflicted to dance. When, however, he stopped to listen and learn the rest of the piece, the dancer helplessly collapsed to the ground, like a marionette attached to his violin strings (Katner 1956: 19–22; De Martino 2005: 93).

In pursuit of alleviation, the afflicted were said to resort to the sounds (*ricorrevano ai suoni*), or to take up the sound (*prendevano il suono*), while musicians were said to make the sign (*facevano il segno*) with their instruments. Sensual stimuli worked to heighten the tarantata's perceptivity. Popular belief states that the tarantate physically became their afflicting spirit and direct bodily experience affirmed this reality, even if of a different order from that of everyday life.

> It is above all necessary to mimic the dance of the little spider – the tarantella. Following an irresistible identification, it is necessary to dance with the spider, indeed be the dancing spider; but at the same time it is necessary to make an actual agonistic moment be felt – the superimposition and imposition of one's own choreutic rhythm upon that of the spider, forcing the spider to dance until it is tired, pursuing it as it flees the chasing foot, or squashing it and stamping it as the foot violently beats the floor to the rhythm of the tarantella. The *tarantato* executes the dance of the little *taranta* (the tarantella) as a victim possessed by the beast and as the hero who subdues the beast by dancing. (De Martino 2005: 36)

De Martino portrays the dancing tarantata as both victim and hero experiencing the ambiguous powers of the spider and St Paul, both credited with the ability to curse and cure. The initial embodiment of or union with the spirit counterparts may have enhanced and aggravated the tarantate's experience of themselves as passive victims, as subjected to the bodily symptoms, social pressures and life conditions afflicting them. Ritual enactment implied surrendering the self. A sacrifice was involved, readiness to give in and let go, 'to allow the tarantula to take over'. The spider allowed for the expression of that which could not be expressed otherwise. It provided a door to new experiences, including the embodiment of a heroine or hero.

In effect, little information is available on how the tarantate experienced rituals, as many claimed that they did not remember what had happened, perhaps tongue-tied by difficulties of verbalizing their experiences or by feelings of being fenced in by social taboos. Moreover, not remembering may also be a cultural norm, emphasizing the belief that the spider takes over the afflicted, who, consequently, cannot remember (Lapassade 1996a: 98). Scholars, meanwhile, have frequently interpreted these experiences in terms of trance or ecstasy, just as some participants in contemporary performances do. Considering the frequent uncritical use of these terms, others voice scepticism about their validity, suspecting the strategic functions such claims may serve and bringing questions of authenticity back on stage.

In spite of these reservations, ritual cases suggest that an awareness of aspects of reality and perceptions of the self, alternative or complementary to those of the afflicted role, were accessed. With the ritual perimeter acting as an experimental playground, the perceived choice of costumes delimitating the tarantate's life to date was stretched to include new self-perceptions, such as a sense of the self as entailing authority and the ability to act and choose. Similarly, contemporary 'magic' circles may bring out little-known aspects of the self, as the accounts of Ada, Tanya and others suggest. Although such 'magical' dynamics are likely to be experienced in diverse and contradictory ways, new experiences of the self may surface as participants tune into and abandon themselves to rhythms synchronized with others and their social and natural surroundings.

Rhythmic Intervention: Choosing to Entrain

The notion of rhythm brings into play conflicting definitions and numerous associations.[7] It may be seen to refer to something greater than any one individual, which, at the same time, may become embodied or physically manifest in any one person. In the context of the tarantula's music and dance, a look at rhythm proposes a view of well-being as grounded in an individual's ability to become ever more

193

aware of rhythmic dimensions and to move beyond automatic, reflexive reactions to these, to the choice of whether, to what degree and in what way to engage with a specific rhythm.

In tarantism rituals recovery was promoted by performance techniques linked both to the physiological rhythms of the afflicted and the existing social and natural cycles of the day-to-day environment. Nowadays, pizzica rhythms may be seen as indicative of social changes, though others dispute its links to daily life (Gala 2002b: 47). Manifold contradictory views and tendencies intertwine as daily and performative rhythms reciprocally shape or contest each other, negotiating identities and perceptions of reality.

As with music, daily performance relies on the continual negotiation and creation of rhythm, 'a future-oriented temporal order … an activity (and action) that anticipates, expects or demands something to come' (You 1994: 363–64). Rhythmic repetition entails an expectation of that which is familiar and, at the same time, the possibility of something different emerging. 'The act of repeating or mirroring highlights the disjuncture between what is shared (mimesis) and what differs (alterity)', as it 'moves through old (repeatedly revisited) yet new (always encountered differently) territory' (Roseman 2002: 125).

This ambivalence is also embodied in the pizzica's ambiguous rhythm. According to Diego Carpitella (in De Martino 2005: 299), the dual nature of the pizzica tarantata, characterized by its beat/offbeat structure, reflected two typical instances of religious healing techniques: the crisis was both accentuated through the impact of the musical offbeat and controlled by the obstinate and constant beat. A similar effect may be provoked through the interrelationship of the tambourine's insistent beat and the melodic tunes of other instruments, such as the violin.[8]

In this way, as one musician confirms, the chaotic experience of tarantism crises could be directed, channelled and transformed: 'There are the cymbals, which take you to the beyond, they give you access to another world. But the constant beat of the tambourine remains. It ensures that you remain linked to the here and now. It reassures you that you won't be left alone, that you are safe and able to come back.'[9] Luisa del Giudice (2005: 249), meanwhile, points to an alternative feminist interpretation, arguing 'that the noise allows the tarantata's world-view to prevail temporarily, with its new and subverted sense of "order", while the steady beat recalls her back to duty and patriarchal "order" – that is the very cause and substance of her *disorder* and *existential chaos*'. In fact, the modern tarantata Tanya emphasized that the state she found herself in when painting to the pizzica didn't leave her feeling unwell but was unsustainable if she wanted to be part of society at large. However such experiences may be lived and interpreted, what is clear is that the direct experience of accessing a dimension understood as other than that of everyday life appeared to be of fundamental importance.[10]

'The power of the rhythmic message within the group,' writes Edward Hall (1983: 184), 'is as strong as anything I know. It is one of the basic components in the process of identification, a hidden force that, like gravity, holds groups together.' Rhythm accentuates not only who is in but also who is out of synchrony, a point taken to heart by the *Sonaglierus Metronomicus* (or circle leader) – as specified by Francesco Patruno (2003) in his list of contemporary piSSica types – 'who claims to direct, in the manner of von Karajan,[11] forty tambourine players, to make them all synchronize, by shouting TEMPOOO when he hears one of the players deviating by 1/32'. Patruno adds that this 'species' of the *Sonaglierus Metronomicus* is 'on the road to extinction – by heart attack'.

Beyond von Karajanesque efforts, the manipulation or conscious use of rhythm entails power, giving or quenching vitality.[12] Human beings, like all other organisms, perform according to internal rhythms, which regulate such automatic body functions as the heartbeat, respiration, circulation and metabolism. At the same time, human interaction relies on an awareness of rhythm and the ability to entrain, to 'become engaged in each other's rhythms' (Hall 1983: 177). As a phenomenon of resonance, entrainment implies the tendency of two oscillating bodies or two or more rhythmic cycles to lock into phase, to vibrate in synchrony. It creates connections – invisible ties between seemingly separate entities.

Performance techniques render such rhythms tangible, sensitizing actors to their subtle influence and fine-tuning skills for perceiving these rhythms. 'An actor should be like a ping-pong player,' says drama therapist Steve Mitchell (1998: 6), 'the attention is following the rhythm of the game, but at the same time is witnessing the process and by so doing is able to take notice of an unexpected possibility'. An awareness of this realm of possibilities implies an openness to new opportunities and a perception of the self as exposed to an abundance of creative possibilities. These may include incorporating fixed victim mentalities, previously seen to poison and limit life circumstances, into a spectrum of diverse roles and rhythms, including those of the 'choreographer' moving flexibly from role to role and rhythm to rhythm.

Vibrating the Spider's Web: Tapping a Source of Vitality

One such role may involve accessing visceral experiences associated with the sensual, sexual, erotic or orgasmic. Cases of tarantism were often linked to forbidden or lost love, as the story of Maria of Nardò indicates. The ritual itself abounded with erotic associations. Sexual taboos and conventions were put aside. The spider was given full lease. Social boundaries were transgressed, cultural limitations overcome. Such experiences in which everyday disjunctures may be seen to dissolve – of which the spider's liminal, transgressive and ambiguous nature appears but a preview – may be reminiscent of religious experiences that contrast 'finite humanity and its bodily limitations with a sense of the infinite and supernatural possibility' (Harris 2000: 306–13). These considerations draw attention to how sexual associations and images are woven into historical and contemporary spider dances and what resonances these may have.

Damian Walter points out that the performative cycle of the pizzica (the slow beginning, increasing activity and rhythm, 'orgasmic' experiences and a subsequent period of cooling down or rest), both in past rituals and some contemporary settings, may be seen to mirror coital and post-coital activity, suggesting parallels between the experience (or sexual arousal) of individual participants and the communal structure of the pizzica itself. From this perspective, even those participants who do not speak of so-called altered states of consciousness may be affected by the communal, intimate and rhythmic interaction of (shared and metaphorical) sexual activity, tying in with ideas of the potentially beneficial and therapeutic qualities of rhythmic experience in broader terms.[13]

'Tarantism is also about sexual issues,' a psychiatrist at the Centre of Mental Health in Lecce confirms. 'In some public performances female tarantate chose a man they found particularly attractive in the crowd and threw themselves at him.'[14] Maurizio Nocera adds: 'Those affected by tarantism are generally troubled in their sexuality. Male tarantati have a tendency to be more feminine and female tarantate tend to be very masculine.'[15] He suggests that in many cases latent homosexual tendencies may have been at the heart of the matter, and equates tarantism with *la sofferenza pelvica*, pelvic suffering:

> This suffering comes from a spider that continues to aggravate its prey. It sets out in the pelvic zone, where the spider moves without the person being conscious of it. Although difficult to verify, it appears that this paroxysmal movement drives the tarantata to auto-produce an uncontrollable orgasmic release. This need for release is not satisfied by making love and only becomes worse doing so. Only song, music, the demand for grace, for a symbol, can calm and tranquillize this need.[16]

Nocera draws an analogy between such paroxysmal movements, in the sense of spasmic contractions typical of an orgasmic climax, and the vibrations of a spider on its web in moments of crisis or death. This point also recalls allusions to sexual intercourse evoked by the tarantate's ritual moves while prostrate on the floor, the erotic connotations of lyrics, as well as the tarantate's designation as St Paul's brides.

Receiving grace, too, has been interpreted in terms of an orgasmic experience. When asked how she experiences this moment, Maria of Nardò responded: 'Ma, che devo dire, si sciolgono le acque'. (But, what can I say, the waters are released) (Mingozzi 1982). This expression, Nocera explains, may refer either to the release of sexual tensions or, taken more literally, to the act of urinating, once again drawing a link to the role of fluids crossing bodily boundaries in healing contexts.[17] Other tarantate specified how they had to 'release water' on entering Galatina, just as Evelina must urinate behind St Paul's altar during her annual pilgrimage.

Some of the tarantate's symptoms (fainting spells and dizziness), as well as the dramatic techniques used (running in a circle or pirouetting), Nocera continues, involve a loss of control and a sense of surrender often seen to characterize orgasmic experiences. Such accounts suggest that a source of gratification and fulfilment, often denied in everyday life, was tapped through performance. In fact, Sandra Gilbert (1986: xi-xii) speaks of the tarantate's dances as 'an interlude of orgasmic freedom': 'The illness or "anomaly" of womanhood in a culture governed by the invisible but many-legged tarantula of patriarchal law takes multiple forms, but its one energy derives from the singular return of the repressed.' Although this view presents women one-sidedly as sexually inhibited and as mere victims to male dominance, it places spider rituals in a celebratory light: evoked as a moment of respite in which the 'true nature' of the tarantate surfaced, rupturing constraints and releasing passions.

Some tarantate were reported to abstain from sex and food prior to the repetition of their rituals (Epifanio Ferdinando in De Martino 2005: 111). Both spheres, food and sex, serve as obvious sites of cultural anxiety, considering particularly the harsh living conditions in the Salento in bygone times, and resonate, moreover, with concerns for bodily boundaries (through food intake, excretion, sexual intercourse or childbirth).

Nowadays, life in the Salento is less physically demanding, but both food and sexuality provide potent spheres of symbolic activity. Experiences of dancing the pizzica today are still frequently linked to questions of sexuality (and associated assumptions), and the pizzica pizzica, too, continues to be a very public expression of sensuality (Chiriatti and Lapassade 1985; Gala 2002a, b; Nocera 2005). According to Daniele Durante (1999: 174), the tambourine's role is influential in this respect. Its constant beat, he argues, stimulates the lower part of the listener's body, leading at times even to sexual arousal. Others link their experience of the pizzica to experiences of sexuality as well. Fernando Bevilacqua recounts:

> It was at a festival, I was playing the tambourine and I realized that a woman began responding with her tambourine. This exchange between us became stronger and stronger, completely absorbing me. Everything around me disappeared, leaving only her and me. Then I found myself high up. She'd lifted me up. I saw her and myself from above. We were united. It was a very strong sensation, like an orgasm.'[18]

Similarly, passionate Salentine dancer and film director Edoardo Winspeare (Nacci 2004: 31) says:

> Personally ... I was cured from my afflictions through the pizzica and through my type of tarantism. I danced a great deal, three to four hours a day, and discovered a lot of things about myself. I discovered my animal side in the pizzica ritual, in the circle ... when I danced with a woman, I rediscovered my masculine side with respect to a female being; the ritual controlled everything and in this way unexpected things came up that I

didn't even think I had, seeing as I grew up ... with a very rigid, Catholic education. The pizzica liberated me.

Although we may question what other factors were and are involved, Winspeare directly pinpoints the pizzica as having a curative influence on his life, in the sense that it allowed him to access new experiences, which he identifies as surprising and liberating.

A young woman describes dancing the pizzica along similar lines:

> You allow the music to pass through you, to enter inside and to do what it wants with you. You become an instrument for something else. You are just a channel and everything passes through you ... when it's over you feel great. I could compare it, even if it isn't similar in any way, to the best time you've made love. (Nacci 2004: 55–59)

In this context it is important, however, not to presuppose a universal physiological response to sexual activity, taking into consideration that cultural, gendered and individual understandings of what constitutes an orgasm may differ and, moreover, imply a metaphorical use of sexual imagery, which does not necessarily translate into experiential terms. 'Ecstasy and joy are inseparable from suffering and eroticized pain in most Christian iconography,' Damian Walter suggests.

> In the case of the tarantate isn't it possible to argue that their use of orgasmic imagery is associated as much with the pain of affliction as it is with joyful release, rather than suggesting that it indicates some kind of unconditional (although pleasurable) 'flooding' of the senses? Perhaps describing their experiences in these terms allows them to articulate a more positive and transformational response to the pain of affliction? They might not be able to escape their pain, but they may be able to reshape the way they integrate the experience of pain into their lives.[19]

'Acute pain', writes medical anthropologist Elisabeth Hsu (2005: 84), 'evokes "presence" and alerts one's "sensory attentiveness",' creating an openness to potentially beneficial impacts from the social context. Although the notion of pain is used to describe lived experiences of diverse quality and intensity, acute (as opposed to chronic) pain 'is acute for both the person in pain and those surrounding him or her, and it thus generates synchronicity, a situation in which all participants involved are acutely aware of only one single event and turn their full attention to it' (ibid.: 85). Boundaries between self and other collapse as 'a state of trans-individual fluidity' emerges and a sense of social connectedness is enhanced (ibid.: 87), reminiscent of 'magical' experiences in the context of the tarantula's music and dance, in both past and present contexts.

In this sense, a focus on notions and experiences of sexuality and sensuality, of the erotic and orgasmic, brings individual and social dimensions of spider dances into resonance: '"Boundary loss" is the individual and "feeling they are one" is the collective way of looking at the same thing,' writes William McNeill (1995: 8–9), 'a blurring of self-awareness and the heightening of fellow-feeling with all who share in the dance.'

Integrating Toxins: Connecting Self and Other

Widening our focus from the level of individual experience in performance situations to the broader contexts of everyday life stories and relationships reveals how music making and dancing may provide a means of integrating 'poisons' of all kinds – harsh living conditions, restricting social relations, limiting self-perceptions. This points to the links between the tarantula's music and dance and how participants related and relate to themselves and others.

Through music, dance and the performance of prescribed acts, the tarantato Francesco Greco underwent profound changes in his perceptions of himself, others and reality at large. Whereas prior to ritual intervention he had felt extremely weak, he became capable of doing inexplicable things and eventually recovered to a state of general well-being. Where doctors had discriminated against him as mentally ill, he became accepted as part of a larger community of tarantate (even if as good as virtual at this stage in time). Finally, his belief in his vulnerability to St Paul's anger turned his initial disrespect for religious saints into a deep-seated respect for the apostle. Although circumstances may not have changed, new perspectives and insights led to a greater sense of well-being.

The situation of women, and men, has changed in the Salento since the tarantate danced and screamed, but the stories of Ada, Tanya and others reveal that the tarantula's influence is anything but swept under the carpet. Daily lives are cross-cut by limitations of all kinds – economic, social, political, as well as bodily – marked by views of the self as having little choice, as being subject to the whims of life circumstances, others' desires or destiny.

In the Salento, as in much of southern Italy, high unemployment figures and low social security combine with little, if any, state support for those without work, for single parents or for the care of children or the elderly.[20] Many Salentines have grown up in such precarious conditions and are adept in finding strategies to cope on a day-to-day basis. Inevitably, family networks play a central role in this context, as do the supplements for daily needs provided by small farm subsistence run by many families in the rural areas. Likewise, young people are frequently restrained by financial restrictions from moving out to live on their own. Those who do may still eat at home, both to be part of family life and in order to live on limited incomes.

Such interdependence may, among other factors, accentuate other prevalent limitations, such as those associated with gender relations. At Torrepaduli, on 15 August 2005, I asked the middle-aged wife of a musician beating his tambourine whether she would like to dance with me. She declined, and after a moment of hesitation explained: 'Poi lui mi fa storie' (Afterwards he makes a fuss).'[21] Her husband's potential reaction limited her moves, holding her in its clutches. This reaction appears to reflect a much more widespread tendency, as Luisa Del Giudice (2005: 250–51) notes:

> Few women hold prominent musical roles today. One finds few women on concert stages, other than in supporting roles (or as the 'pretty face', that is, the singer in the ensemble). '*Stanno lì … con le mani legate*' (There they stand … with their hands tied), laments one female musician. They continue, however, to constitute the majority of dancers on the public piazzas, but they are surprisingly absent as cultural activists.

Slowly, this is changing, with a few female singers, such as Imma Giannuzzi, Enza Pagliara and Cinzia Villani, leading their own bands.

Nevertheless, the predominantly restrictive roles of women in the pizzica world may be seen as representative of women's roles more generally. In the Salento, a nineteen-year-old girl from the small town of Uggiano La Chiesa has to be home by 11 p.m. at the latest to keep to her father's terms. Another Salentine woman in her mid-thirties tells me of her difficult relationship with her father and how this has limited her life. 'Now I'm catching up on the lost years. I've learnt through suffering,' she says with tears in her eyes. 'Now I'm travelling, studying, walking on my own feet.'[22] Only recently, it seems, has she cut through the fine threads of her own attitudes and belief systems – no doubt shaped by guilt, duty, fear, economic dependence, as well as social pressures – stepping out of her familiar inculcated sense of self and its limitations and, making her own decisions, moving into territory that she had not previously dared tiptoe into, while inevitably jeopardizing existing family relations.

But men, it appears, are no less entangled. A Salentine medic gives me his view, influenced by Jungian ideas:

> Tarantism is linked to a regionally specific collective unconscious and culturally specific archetypes: these women weave their webs around men, entangling them. Men know they will become their victims. They already have this propensity seeing that *il mammismo* is so widely diffused. Mothers' hold on men is extremely strong in this region and from their mothers' hands they pass into their women's hold.[23]

Another middle-aged man asserts:

> For me a woman is a spider. To tell the truth, once I was looking for the ideal woman, but on my way I only met women as spiders. When I say ideal woman, I'm alluding to the knowing woman, one who is able to understand me, to tolerate me too. But, as I said before, I haven't been lucky: on my way I have always found spiders. (Nocera 2005: 62)

An implicit analogy with the myth of the female tarantula eating its male partner after copulating springs to mind: the opposite sex as temptation and condemnation combined, reminiscent of assumptions about women, primitivism and sexuality more generally: of how 'entomologists' anthropomorphizing descriptions of love affairs of praying mantises and black widow spiders had proven to be directly analogous to the effects of the sexual woman's depredations in the human environment' (Dijkstra 1996: 212–13).

What emerges from both male and female accounts about gender relations is a game of victims and tyrants, a sense of the self as falling prey to the demands and expectations of those onto whom the label of tyrants is projected. Such relations inevitably bring into play the problematic and controversial debates on 'honour and shame' in the Mediterranean context, distinguishing, in basic terms, divisions of labour and morality according to gender (Goddard 1987, 1996; Giordano 2002). Such relations, moreover, risk promoting assumptions of male and female as clear-cut categories based on a specific gender model. Both men and women use the idiom of tarantism to convey feelings of being helpless, powerless and at the mercy of marionette strings pulled by others, whereas multiple gender discourses and categories, conflicting and contradicting each other, are likely to be at hand (Moore 1994: 824). In this sense, it becomes vital to attend to the 'multiple perspectives, shifting purposes and reflexive and ironic commentaries' (Raheja and Gold 1994: 9) among women, as well as men, that challenge normalizing and essentializing discourses.

In fact, the tarantula's music and dance have increasingly turned into symbols of self-assertion, power and celebration.

> The music of *tarantismo* has been recast as a celebratory practice of current Salentine identity. It follows that the figure of the tarantata has also been positively recast. Not only has the stigma been lifted from the tarantata's shoulders, there seems to be a growing positive reevaluation (romanticization? glorification?) of this figure as it undergoes something of an apotheosis. She has become a heroine, passing from something of a feared outcast to shaman. Possessed by a spider god with whom she becomes one, temporarily unbound by societal norms, she explores the existential fringe via the dance, bringing spiritual and mental health back to herself and to the community (which is literally standing around her). She is not merely a passive receptor of musical vibrations that others played to awaken her, therefore, but a spiritual leader, acting on behalf of those incapable (though just as needy) of freeing themselves. (Del Giudice 2005: 253–54)

Ada Metafune, for example, gives workshops on the tarantula's music and dance in the Salento and throughout Italy and, at times, finds herself transmitting her personal experiences to course participants confronting her with problematic aspects of their lives, sensing the insights and strength she has gained from her own life crises. In this sense, women such as Ada may come to embody role models for others, testifying to possibilities of transforming perceptions of the self, from 'powerless' to 'empowered', from 'helpless victim' to 'creative choreographer'. Clearly, however, such views equally risk presenting essentialized categories, which are likely not only to coexist and overlap, but also to shift among infinite subtle nuances between these categories, as well as unforeseen possibilities.

Zooming out yet further from the impact of the tarantula's music and dance on individual life stories and relations draws attention to the collective influence – and inherent risks – of this music and dance on local discourses on identity.

Transforming Identities: Evoking a Sense of Belonging

'We have it inside' is a frequently voiced stance, suggesting that the pizzica and everything associated with it is 'pulsing' in the blood of those born in the Salento, creating a sense of identity commonly, unreflectively, voiced in the expression 'We're DOC Salentines!' DOC, *denominazione d'origine controllata*, controlled denomination of origin, is the unit of measure and quality assigned to regionally specific products of the European Union and ascribed to the people of the Salento as a (perceived) guarantee of originality, as an official stamp of legitimacy. In this sense, the tarantula and the pizzica pay lip service to social constructions of local identity voiced with enthusiasm, becoming almost an expression of modesty, as the ability to perform is ultimately seen as a heaven-sent gift not attributed to individual talent, commitment or merit. Yet the criteria that make one person DOC but not another are rarely clear, as the rhythm of the pizzica is essentialized into a biological function, naturalized and, inevitably, mystified.

'If in the fifties and sixties tourist invitations to the Salento tended to ignore, even hide the last "relics" of tarantism, today the same invites express pride with reference to tarantism: come to the land of tarantism … come to know the Salento, it has tarantism, with its antique, Dionysian and perhaps even pre-Greek roots, in its blood,' writes social anthropologist Paolo Apolito (2000: 140). He stresses how the myth of the tarantula has taken on religious qualities, all the more potent as this myth is not, like many others, delocalized but has, instead, been reinvented within the region of its apparent origins. Such a focus on what is perceived as 'local' can be observed across Europe, and may be viewed not only as a counter-reaction to 'globalization', but also as a result of European funding incentives for regional as opposed to national initiatives, aiming to promote associations with a united Europe of regions beyond national affiliations. The Salentine peninsula more specifically is a roulette wheel of potential identities and fleeting points of reference, having been exposed to a history of foreign domination and becoming a major gateway to Europe for refugees and asylum seekers in recent years, as well as a newly prized tourist oasis and sought-after region for northern Europeans seeking to buy a holiday or retirement home.

In the past, victims of the tarantula naturalized their afflictions through spider poisoning and the tarantate were often severely criticized for manipulating this link for personal and political reasons. In the contemporary Salento, too, musicians and dancers, as well as cultural administrators and intellectuals, are frequently accused of wanting to enlarge their own name or bank account, of exploiting the tarantula's music and dance for manipulative purposes. Clearly, other issues are at stake.

In recent years, social anthropologist Giovanni Pizza (2002a, b) has contributed significantly to a critical discourse on questions of essentialized and naturalized identities in the Salento. He writes: 'Only the conscious or unconscious incorporation of hegemonic stereotypes, even if widespread among the population, can incite us to consider our sense of belonging to be inscribed in our blood, our flesh or even in our genetic inheritance' (2002a: 55). He repeatedly warns against the passive incorporation of platitudes inseparable from existing power structures and ideologies. The pizzica exacerbates sensations, beliefs, attitudes and opinions, making them more acute, amplifying the intentions with which it is performed, acting as hi-fi systems for enacted beliefs and motivations. Voices, instruments, microphones, not to speak of satellite television, propagate rivalry and ambitions of becoming the latest star on stage just as much as gestures of solidarity and friendship. Every actor in this game faces the choice of whether or not to use whatever the pizzica brings to the surface as a 'methodological and ethical mirror metaphor' (Pizza 2002a: 53).

> The rhetoric of conserving one's own identity often hides not the fear of looking at 'the other', but the fear of looking into one's own face ... out of fear of reflecting oneself ... of finding oneself in front of the recurrence of a monstrous image ... Obscuring the mirror is a precondition for an essentialist discourse that conceives identity as objects, essences to preserve 'intimate' and 'profound' truths; it is a political operation of concealing motivations, intentions and the objectives of one's own discourses and actions. (ibid.: 52)

Obscuring potential mirrors of self-reflection may provoke automatic reflexes to project onto 'others' (groups, individuals, bodies) everything the self is not identified with, that which is rejected and condemned, making personal 'demons' visible in an amplified, tangible form. What is more, every minimal glimpse of this mirror may create a further reaction of grasping yet more strongly onto that which is accepted as part of the self's identity, that which is seen as agreeable and amenable, including naturalizing explanations diagnosing pizzica rhythms in bloodstreams and DNA codes.

With regard to southern Italy these issues have been widely discussed in terms of the 'Southern Question', attesting to the deeply rooted differences between Italy's northern and southern regions (Schneider 1998). In his historical study of ritual cycles in the town of Calvello in Basilicata, Hermann Tak (2000: 243) stresses how '"the North" became an imaginary "other" replacing one time fierce antagonistic inter-town relations'. Such juxtapositions also emerge in Christian Giordano's (1992) discussion of a 'culture of superimposition' characterizing regions such as southern Italy, subjected to hundreds of years of domination by foreign powers, resulting in the internalization of fatalistic attitudes such as the 'image of *miseria*', a belief in poverty as collective fate, or the *governo ladro* (thieving government), involving perceptions of the state as hostile and unreliable. Although these concepts need to be taken on with care, cultural self-reification or essentialism in the context of the tarantula's music and dance today is likely to be a way of reaffirming one's values in the face of these broader socio-economic power structures.[24]

With these considerations in mind, individual experiences of performance situations inevitably mould and are moulded by social relations activated in these contexts, as well as intentions and interpretations that encourage or inhibit participation. As these pages reveal, the tarantula's music and dance hold the potential not only to accentuate individual afflictions and social conflicts but also to promote well-being and the reintegration of individuals in the larger webs of everyday community lives. As a creative platform for new experiences and perceptions, they hold the power both to exclude and include other potential participants. They may deepen situations and sensations of disjuncture just as much as those of belonging.

In the past, identification with the toxic spider was facilitated through music and dance, as well as such sensual stimuli as scents and colours. This provided a basis for transformations (without any guarantee, however), integrating the spider, and all rejected aspects of the self it had come to embody, into a new, broader sense of the self. In the same way, a confrontation with what is seen to be the 'perpetrator' today – be it globalization, the Italian state, foreign musical directors, other music groups, the opposite sex or dismissed desires – may provide a first step towards transformation.

As music is allowed to take over, the familiar and foreign may be expressed and brought into communication, linking the self and other and evoking a sense of belonging to humanity at large. Fatalistic perceptions of the self as victim become redundant, and ever more choices are created as additional outfits are integrated into existing costume cupboards. What is fundamental to the recovery of well-being, vitality and presence is the way of performing and underlying intent – of finding the 'right air', its magical dimensions and potential to rhythmically intervene – and whether these are integrated and interpreted to either perpetuate or transform afflicting self-perceptions. In this sense, spider dances today continue to entail both golden cages and the keys to these.

Notes

1. See Fernando Bevilacqua's (1995) video clip *Stretti nello spazio senza tempo*, Tight in Space without Time, which aims to convey experiences of the tarantula's music and dance in visual terms.
2. An interesting link may also be drawn here to the use of circles as an ancient magical formula (Dauterman Maguire et al. 1989).
3. Alessano, 10 August 2005.
4. Ostuni, 22 February 2008.
5. Casarano, 29 May 1998.
6. The English word choreutic, Dorothy Zinn explains, is a translation of 'the term *coreutico*, from the Italian noun *coreutica* – the art of dance' (in De Martino 2005: 29).
7. 'There is not, and perhaps will never be a "precise and generally accepted definition" of the term rhythm,' writes Haili You (1994: 373), if we consider rhythm as a category of human experience or mode of being (ibid.: 374). Musicologists contradict such a relativist stance and, despite changing definitions through time and disagreements in etymological foundations, tend to define 'duration and stress, constructions in time and gradations in strength' as its constituent features (Sadie 1980: 805).
8. Marina Roseman (2002: 125) observes similarities in Temiar music generated by bamboo-tube stampers: 'The sense of sameness yet *différence*, embodied in the repetition and alteration of the continual tube beats, sets the stage sensorially for heightened relationships between familiarity and strangeness ... This space is performatively constructed not only through the tube-beats' relationship to one another, but through the relationship between constantly duple-rhythmed percussion, on one hand, and changing melodies, on the other.'
9. Cisternino, 3 May 1998.
10. This also relates to Carol Laderman's (1981: 488) reference to a 'rich order' in her discussion of the empirical reality of symbolic systems of food avoidances among the Temiar in Malaysia: 'The dynamic nature of these symbolic systems provides a structure for the logical working out of individual variability reminiscent of the musical structure of a chaconne. Although the ground bass repeats endlessly through the piece ... the upper voices weave variation after variation above it. The effect is that of rich order, rather than either chaos or stasis.'
11. Austrian conductor Herbert von Karajan (1908–89).
12. Pierre Bourdieu (1977: 7) refers to the rhythms of society and politics in his theory of practice relative to the manipulation of time: '"Synchronization" of a social action not only reflects the collective spatio-temporal representations but also maintains the symbolic order and revitalizes the

social existence of the group itself ... There is unlimited scope for strategies exploiting the possibilities offered by the manipulation of the tempo of action – holding back or putting off, maintaining suspense or expectation, or on the other hand, hurrying, hustling, surprising and stealing a march, not to mention the art of ostentatiously giving time ("devoting one's time to someone") or withholding it ("no time to spare").'

13. Damian Walter, personal communication.
14. Lecce, 1 April 1998.
15. Lecce, 24 November 1997.
16. Lecce, 4 June 1998.
17. Lecce, 6 July 1999.
18. Galatina, 24 June 1999.
19. Personal communication.
20. In 2001, unemployment in the Salento was at 17% among men and 27.9% among women, as opposed to a national average of 11.58% (http://dawinci.istat.it/MD/). Meanwhile, many businesses continue not to declare their workers because of high social benefit costs and, in 2007, salaries were as low as 25 euros per day for an eight-hour bar shift or 500 euros or less per month (for secretarial or factory jobs).
21. Torrepaduli, 15 August 2005.
22. Lecce, 10 November 2005.
23. Lecce, 24 August 2005. The speaker refers to the overprotective tendencies characterizing mother-son relationships, particularly in southern Italy, with men (and women) continuing to live in their parents' homes well into middle age and beyond, unless they marry and set up a household of their own.
24. I thank Susanne Wessendorf for bringing Giordano's work to my attention.

Part IV
Conclusion

In this final section, I draw together the threads that emerged in the foregoing chapters, in order to return to the key questions that have directed this study: how has the tarantula's dance changed over time and what does it reveal about the link between performance practices and well-being? Major differences between past and present dances have been spotlighted in preceding chapters while at the same time bringing to light a common thread: the need to find the 'right thread or air' and the intention of surrendering to it. Looking at this further, the notions of rhythm and entrainment have emerged as possible indicators linking experiences of well-being and performance, as have processes of identification and integration, as well as the ability to recognize the origins of conflict in day-to-day attitudes and behaviour. Although this study may focus only on a small proportion of those engaging with the tarantula's music and dance today, these features show how the individual experience of performance practices can provide a learning ground for choices furthering well-being, in the sense of vitality and presence.

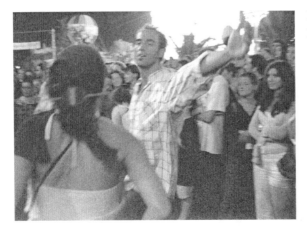

Fig. 9.1 The pizzica pizzica, Torrepaduli, 15 August 1999 (photo: Karen Lüdtke).

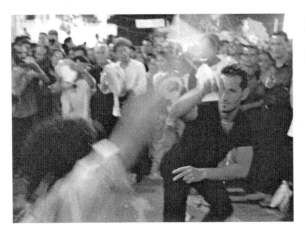

Fig. 9.2 The scherma, Torrepaduli, 15 August 1999 (photo: Karen Lüdtke).

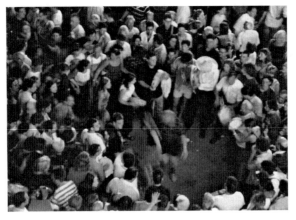

Fig. 9.3 A circle of dancers, musicians and spectators at the festival of St Rocco, Torrepaduli, 15 August 1999 (photo: Karen Lüdtke).

Chapter 9
Dancing Beyond Spiders

> Rhythm is the most perceptible
> and least material thing.
>
> John Chernoff (1981: 23)

Evelina's Story: Living with the Tarantula

In August 2005, together with my Salentine friend Patrizia, I arrive once more at Evelina's homestead. Walking into the courtyard through the main gate, we see her standing, tiny and delicate, no more than one metre twenty tall, framed by a pointed archway leading to the stables. She greets us from a distance, with a firm, warm voice: 'Ciao!' and, recognizing who we are, raises one hand in a joking, chiding gesture. We kiss the cheeks of her beaming face in greeting. She is eighty-one years old now and her back curves at the shoulders, but her eyes and stride are full of vitality. She takes us to see the cows, chickens and pigs in their stalls and then invites us to come through to greet Michela, her daughter-in-law, *la padrona di casa*, the landlady, as she says, taking herself out of the way, almost erasing herself with this gesture, small as she is, seemingly unaware that it was her we had primarily come to see.

We greet Michela and, while she finishes what she was doing, sit and talk with Evelina. Her story pours forth in significant episodes as she speaks in dialect to my friend Patrizia. She tells about the death of her father when she was just twelve and the loss, soon after, of her brother killed in the war, a letter arriving to announce his death. Over the years she has often told me about them, eager to communicate these incisive snapshots of her life.

Michela joins us and begins to take over the conversation. Others come too: two of Michela's children, neighbours, friends, mainly elderly. Most I know from my initial period of fieldwork (1997–98) when I joined them on several occasions to pick tobacco in their fields. Now, seven years later, memories come up of those times; jokes told then, people passed away since. At this point, Evelina no longer goes into the fields. At the time, she kept up better than I could with the fast-moving group of harvesters, stripping the large, oily leaves off their strong stalks, creating cracking sounds that mixed with the chit-chat and banter linking the group partly hidden from one another behind the head-high plants. Michela has stopped working in the fields, too. She hopes to receive a disability pension due to her back and leg problems, and to run only the big house and adjoining bed and breakfast on her own, now that all of her children work in the north of Italy for most of the year.

We sit and chat. Only Evelina is silent. She has almost become invisible with the back and forth of words and laughter, raising the sound level in the room, flying over her head. Others answer questions posed to her. She seems to have lost her voice as she sits, sunken away, though aware of what is going on. I am struck by the way her bubbly personality is tucked away within this larger group of people. She stands out not only for her age and wiry, energetic body, but also for her lack of frills in both manner and dress. 'Per la nonna (for Gran), there's no such thing as fashion,' her grandson points out affectionately, and Michela adds that Evelina has insisted on wearing a black dress, headscarf, socks and long sleeves ever since the day her mother died. There was no way of persuading her to roll up her sleeves, even in the hot summer months. She is so different, Patrizia remarks later, from the southern Italian image of femininity and the elderly women around her, with their permed and propped-up short hair, rounded figures and concerned gossip.

Michela tells how she had always felt that Evelina was extremely sensitive and had let her be to do her own thing, so as not to aggravate her condition or cause her to suffer and fall prey to yet another crisis. She tells how now she is tied to the house, not wanting to leave Evelina alone, as she has refused to leave the perimeter of their homestead ever since she fainted in their village church some years back.

Chained to each other by the implications of crisis and care, Evelina and Michela share one rooftop, one family destiny: Evelina's mother had remarried and their move to the current homestead was marked by the jealousy of others. Evelina had given birth to her son, Roberto, out of wedlock, precluding any future marriage, falling into the socially and religiously defined sin of being a single mother, cutting through social taboos and expectations of the time, and even of today. No wonder the tarantula had found her.

Michela had married into this entanglement. Once married to Roberto, she had moved in with him, Evelina and her mother. Her life has been one of hard work and dedication to the family. Her early pension on the basis of physical disabilities seems likely to be linked to all this. Every year she has accompanied her mother-in-law to Galatina, together with her husband and, later, her youngest son, Paolo, named after the fateful saint holding the strings of her mother-in-law's life. Paolo's name was a promise fulfilled to the apostle when Evelina was in the claws of extreme crisis. Michela, pregnant at the time, made a vow to name her child after the saint if Evelina lived and returned to being well.

Evelina's family make no fuss about their fate. *La nonna*, Evelina, is treated with the affection she radiates to others. Yet, when I ask whether they would consider telling their story, Michela and her daughter's reaction is a firm, choral 'No!' 'She will only start to cry,' Michela explains, and her daughter, now in her late twenties, adds, referring to her mother and grandmother: 'I'd prefer not to speak about these things, especially if they're things of the past. It's better to let them be, especially for them.' There is no wish to stir up deep waters and, instead, everything possible is done to maintain the delicate status quo.

Clearly, this family has come to terms with its lot in the form of a frail balance within the tarantula's web, governed by the tarantula and requiring constant care and compromises. At times it holds Evelina in its claws, turning her into a protagonist on St Paul's 'stage' in Galatina, putting the whole family into gear to fulfil its whims. At other times it pushes Evelina into invisibility and silence, letting the family take over, speaking for her in disregard of her physical presence.

As Patrizia and I leave, with gifts of home-grown vegetables, eggs and home-made cheese, we greet Roberto, busy milking the cows. Michela says she will go and help him now, as she hadn't been able to assist him during our visit. Earlier he had passed by briefly, welcoming us warmly and cordially but without stopping in his tracks to continue his afternoon chores. He has always struck me as a silent and hard worker.

As we drive home I cannot help but think that although no dance, music or straightforward curative rituals are involved in Evelina's life story, there is a subtle play at hand: a pendulum swinging between the extremes of all-controlling domination by her tarantula through the crises it is seen to provoke, with Evelina's family playing to its tunes, and self-annihilating surrender, with Evelina giving herself up to the orchestrations of her family. In the chapel of St Paul, I have seen Evelina collapse and her body turn rigid, immobile, frozen. In a social context in her home, surrounded by family and friends, I see her fall into a state of 'absence', her presence withdrawn, her participation reduced to zero. Yet, at other moments, her vibrant and sensitive presence radiates to everyone present. Such pendulum swings may be seen to have characterized the lives of the tarantate more generally.

Tarantula Rhythms: Reflections on Performance and Well-being

Historical documents reveal how the tarantate's crises have always been marked by symptoms oscillating between the extremes of hyperactivity and lethargy. Their stories, meanwhile, reveal discordant relations with others and the social context at large. Rhythms of breath, pulse and motion snapped and went berserk: bodies became listless, drowsy, paralysed, or were taken over by convulsions, shaking and trembling. Interaction with others and the world around became jarred and handicapped, dictated by taboos and social judgements, as well as variables of pain, anger or fear.

Physiological, as well as social rhythms were thrown out of balance. An infection of the afflicted individual's skin surface and bloodstream was metaphorically linked to an affliction on the level of social relations. Likewise, the cases of some new tarantati, dancing to feel better, are linked to a lack of rhythmic synchronicity, to fractured relationships, feelings of fragmentation, emptiness and a desire for deeper meaning. Leonardo da Vinci's evocative phrase – 'The bite of the *taranta* maintains a man in his intention, that is whatever he was thinking when he was bitten' (cod. H. 18v. in De Martino 2005) – suggests that traumatic experiences associated with the tarantula's bite became inscribed not only in the body, but also in the sense of self, safeguarded ever after, leaving the afflicted individual suspended within the specific perspective or web of meanings activated at the moment of the bite. Time stood still though bodies aged and lives passed. A discrepancy emerged, a sense of the self as no longer linked to the present.

Here performative acts intervened, providing an alternative code. Even in the absence of music and dance, Evelina's tendency to withdraw may be remedied by her public appearance on St Paul's ground, dictated by the tarantula's presence. Here she enters into relational frameworks very different from those of her secluded everyday life. Her family generally seeks to protect her, to cushion the impact, pushing the chapel door closed against the weight of the crowd outside, motivated by a wish for privacy, a desire to get through this unasked-for but unavoidable visit as quickly and as calmly as possible. I have always been struck by their matter-of-fact manner, suggestive of nothing to prove and a lot to accept, their openness to the questions of curious onlookers without overextending themselves. Evelina herself tends to avoid anyone approaching her, but at times, walking with one arm akimbo, appears anything but indifferent to all the attention she receives. Under St Paul's shield she finds her place once a year in a social life outside the self-imposed perimeter of her homestead, taking a step beyond her quotidian limits in the tarantula's name. She surrenders and makes her sacrifice.

My impression is, however, that if Evelina had the choice she would not go to Galatina. If only she could, she would stay at home. Yet she is compelled to visit St Paul's chapel to maintain her delicate equilibrium. Her pilgrimage remains her only way out. Here a fundamental difference emerges from today's tarantati. Those who participate in the tarantula's music and dance with the expressive desire to get better based on previous experiences viewed as beneficial are driven by a choice rather than compulsion: a choice based on the knowledge that the tarantula's music and dance may be one possible avenue to feeling better, a means of letting go, a way of accessing experiences alternative to those provoked by difficult situations their daily lives may entail. In this sense, today's tarantati appear to actively seek out the tarantula and its 'magic' to free themselves from conventions and restrictions in their lives, while Evelina, it seems, if only she knew how, would gladly cut the spider's threads.

Although she gains temporary release through her visits to Galatina, ever since she was first bitten in 1953, over half a century ago, Evelina has never completely recovered. In this sense, her pilgrimages may be seen to be placed at the service of her affliction. Underlying circumstances – including belief systems, social relations and economic conditions – may persist, as do her symptoms. A similar risk of perpetuating afflictions may be equally inherent in attempts at engaging with the tarantula's music and dance to promote well-being today. Dancing and music making may be a way to face 'demons', afflictions and hardship, to express these and come to terms with them, just as they may be a form of distraction, of addiction or compulsion, propagating the means to look away.

This ambiguous nature of spider dances points to key reflections on well-being and performance more generally. It alerts us to the value of taking a sensitive approach to certain human conditions associated with crises, which may be easily dispatched as pathological in contemporary Western society, when in effect they may be inherently transformative and therapeutic if protected and expressed within a socially accepted explanatory and supportive framework. The tarantate were not described as ill. They were seen as normal people under the tarantula's spell. Rituals accentuated their crises. Treatment involved enhancing symptoms, by providing sensual stimuli that provoked crises further. It also relied on containment, allowing for the expression of such crises in a safe environment.

In this sense, symptoms were part and parcel of treatment, an initial expression of the issue at heart, pointing to the potential inherent in acute pain expression in a safe social context. As crises were aggravated a homeopathic process was set in motion. Personal stories and memories could be recomposed and re-conceptualized as new perspectives and experiences of the self emerged through the externalization of symptoms, the expression of crises, and the possibilities of beneficial inputs, such as support, nourishment and containment, from the broader social environment. At the same time, such social frameworks of support could inevitably be exploited or exploitative, thereby perpetuating crises. These inherent risks demand a careful consideration of the intentions motivating any kind of performance.

Spider dances further draw attention to the value of developing a sensitivity towards entrainment and the choice of whether or not to entrain. This challenges conceptions of the boundedness of individual existence in favour of an amplified notion of the self, as being part of and affected by broader societal circumstances, contexts and values.

Rhythm permeates perceived dualities of body and mind, biology and society, self and other, demanding an openness to letting go of perceived boundaries, self-perceptions, views of reality to leave room for the new and unexpected. In performance contexts, this is facilitated not only by a unitary and continuous rhythm, but also by the intensity or emotional input of performers, who, in turn, must be willing to let themselves be transported by the rhythms that emerge. Such surrender is further promoted, when rhythms are recognized and legitimized as socially meaningful, through a link to the socio-natural cycles and performative rhythms of everyday life. Here too, however, underlying intentions are fundamental and the extent to which these allow not only for 'letting go' in a safe environment, but also for reintegration into wider socio-natural webs.

Finally, all the 'arts', as forms of creative expression, provide potentially curative stimuli, creating alternative – imagined and invented – realities. As rules and values of everyday life become redundant, notions of good and evil are suspended and everything becomes possible. Questions of authenticity (whether of crises, states of consciousness or musical execution) may lose their pertinence, as invention, in the sense of performative realities, may become a healing device in itself. Although easily discredited as pretence and not free from risks of manipulation and abuse, invention opens up new possibilities and perspectives, which may be integrated into daily lives if safeguarded by a protective framework. As such, imagined and invented realities provide space for inventions, for creative interventions and discontinuity: room for something alternative, unfamiliar, new to emerge, in the face of claims for continuity, maintaining the status quo of afflicting circumstances.

Dances with spiders suggest that well-being and soundness emerge where the sense of self integrates ever more aspects of existence. In this sense, healing becomes a form of art in itself, and a choice, aimed at evoking new and 'wholesome', if inconsistent and ever-expanding, experiences of the self. Rhythmic performance, meanwhile, reveals itself as one potential means of regaining a sense of the ground under our feet and the sky above our heads, by developing the ability to tune in, with spiders and demons projected elsewhere, in order to draw them, too, into the dance.

Epilogue

On 29 June 2007, around 5.30 a.m., Evelina once again steps into St Paul's chapel in Galatina. She gives a shrill cry, drops back into the prepared arms of her grandson and, as if taken over by shock waves, stamps her feet forcefully onto the ground. My stomach churns. She is lowered to the floor. The chapel is filled to the brim with onlookers. Outside, the pizzica circle, previously blocking the entrance, has stopped resounding across the square. All night long, musicians and dancers had (despite reprimands) selected this location to execute their modern-day vigil, following the concert on the main square of San Pietro piazza the night before.

After a few minutes, Evelina returns to her senses. She disappears briefly behind the altar and is greeted by friendly questions on her return. She answers without hesitation. My eye catches that of her son and we smile at each other: the chit-chat seems to disperse the tension of what had just occurred. As Evelina steps out of the chapel a round of applause greets her. She waves back in acknowledgement. By the year 2007, her crises have propelled her to celebrity. With her family she moves on to the main church, following a route they have taken for over half a century. I accompany them to 'their' pew and for a coffee in the legendary – perhaps aptly named – Eros Bar. As we say goodbye, Evelina lingers behind a little. She has something to tell me: 'Abbiamo fatto pace' (We have made peace).

Bibliography

Agamennone, M. (ed.). 2005. *Musiche tradizionali del Salento: le registrazioni di Diego Carpitella e Ernesto De Martino (1959, 1960)*. Rome: Squilibri.

Almiento, M. 1990. 'Per una visione estetico-antropologico del tarantismo pugliese', Tesi di Laurea. University of Lecce.

———. 1994. 'E Maria continua a ballare', in G. Di Lecce (ed.), *La danza della piccola taranta*. Rome: Sensibili alle foglie, pp. 255–66.

Alvin, J. 1966. *Music Therapy*. London: Baker.

Amit, V. 2002. *Realizing Community: Concepts, Social Relationships and Sentiments*. London: Routledge.

Ampolo, V. and G. Zappatore (eds). 1999. *Musica, droga e transe: materiali di ricerca*. Rome: Sensibili alle foglie.

Antonacci, A. 1988. 'Il tarantolismo degli stenterelli', *Il Galatino*, 14: 1.

Angrisani, M. 2000. 'Tarantolati. Tradizione e innovazione nella cultura salentina contemporanea', Tesi di Laurea. University of Salerno.

Anon. 1967. 'Tarantism, St Paul and the Spider', *Times Literary Supplement*, 27 April.

———. 2002. 'Alla Bua', *quiSalento*, 8,9: 25.

———. 2005. 'La Taranta diventa una "griffe"', *Gazzetta del Mezzogiorno*, 10 August: 10.

———. 2007. 'I ritmi della pizzica del secolo nuovo', *quiSalento*, 15 July – August, 7, 8: 81.

Apolito, P. (ed.). 1994. *Annabella Rossi: Lettere da una tarantata*. Lecce: Argo.

———. 2000. 'Tarantismo, identità locale, postmodernità', in G. Di Mitri (ed.), *Quarant'anni dopo De Martino*. Nardò: Besa, pp. 135–43.

Archetti, E. 1999. *Masculinities: Football, Polo and the Tango in Argentina*. Oxford: Berg.

Ardillo, C. 1997. 'Tarantismo, tarantella, etnorap. Metamorfosi e sincretismi nella cultura del Salento', Tesi di Laurea. University of Bologna.

Artaud, A. 1958. *The Theatre and its Double*. New York: Grove Press.

Arthur, P. 2004. 'I menhir del Salento', in G. Bertelli (ed.), *Puglia Preromanica dal V secolo agli inizi dell'XI*. Milan: Jaca Book, pp. 289–91.

Attanasi, F. 2007. *Le musiche nel tarantismo. Le fonti storiche*. Pisa: Edizioni ETS.

Backman, E. 1952. *Religious Dances in the Christian Church and in Popular Medicine*. London: George Allen and Unwin.

Badone, E. and Roseman, S. 2004. (eds). *Intersecting Journeys: The Anthropology of Pilgrimage and Tourism*. Urbana: University of Illinois Press.

Baglivi, G. [1696] 1999. 'De anatome morsu et effectibus tarantulae', in M. Merico (ed.), *De tarantulae – 1695*, trans. R. Pellegrini. Lecce: Aramirè.

Baldwin, M. 1997. 'Dancing with Spiders: Tarantism in Early Modern Europe', in P. Theerman and K. Parshall (eds), *Experiencing Nature*. Boston: Kluwer Academic Publications, pp. 163–91.

Bandini, G. 2006. *Il bacio della tarantola*. Rome: Newton Compton.

Banfield, E. 1958. *The Moral Basis of a Backward Society*. Chicago: Free Press.

Barba, E. 1995. *The Paper Canoe: a Guide to Theatre Anthropology*. London: Routledge.

——. 2001. 'L'essence du théâtre', in J. Feral (ed.), *Les Chemins de l'acteur*. Quebec: Editions Québec Amérique.

Barba, E. and N. Savarese (eds). 1991. *A Dictionary of Theatre Anthropology: the Secret Art of the Performer*. London: Routledge.

Barbati, C., G. Mingozzi and A. Rossi (eds). 1978. *Profondo Sud: viaggio nei luoghi di Ernesto De Martino a vent'anni da 'Sud e magia'*. Milan: Feltrinelli.

Barone, M. 2006. 'Viaggia la Taranta: gran finale al Carnevale di Venezia', *Quotidiano di Lecce*, 25 February: 29.

Bartholomew, R. 1994. 'Tarantism, Dancing Mania and Demonopathy: the Anthro-political Aspects of "Mass Psychogenic Illness"', *Psychological Medicine*, 24: 281–306.

Basile, A. 2000. *Taranto, taranta, tarantismo*. Taranto: Nuoveproposte.

Basu, P. 2004. 'Route-metaphors of "roots-tourism": the Scottish Highlands', in S. Coleman and J. Eade (eds), *Reframing Pilgrimage: Cultures in Motion*. London: Routledge, pp. 150–74.

Barz, G. and T. Cooley (eds). 1997. *Shadows in the Field: New Perspectives for Fieldwork in Ethnomusicology*. Oxford: Oxford University Press.

Beattie, J. 1977. 'Spirit Mediumship as Theatre', *RAIN*, 20: 1–6.

Becker, J. 2004. *Deep Listeners: Music, Emotion and Trancing*. Bloomington: Indiana University Press.

Beeman, W. 1993. 'The Anthropology of Theatre and Spectacle', *Annual Review of Anthropology*, 22: 369–93.

Bennetts, S. 2006. 'Bitten by Revival Bug: an Ancient Southern Italian Possession Cult is Suddenly Fashionable', *Weekend Australian*, 28 January: R10.

Berkeley, G. [1717] 1979. *Viaggio in Italia*. Naples: E. Jessop and M. Fimiani.

Berman, M. 1990. *Coming to Our Senses: Body and Spirit in the History of the West*. London: Unwin Hyman.

Biagi, L. 2004. 'Spider Dreams: Ritual and Performance in Apulian Tarantismo and Tarantella', Ph.D. thesis. New York University.

Blacking, J. 1976. *How Musical is Man?* London: Faber and Faber.

——. (ed.). 1977. *The Anthropology of the Body*. London: Academic Press.

Blasi, S. 2001. 'I miracoli della taranta', *Quotidiano di Lecce*, 230: 1–8.

Boissevain, J. 1992. *Revitalising European Rituals*. London: Routledge.

Boorstin, D. 1961. *The Image*. New York: Vintage.

Bourdieu, P. 1977. *Outline of a Theory of Practice*. Cambridge: Cambridge University Press.

Bourguignon, E. (ed.). 1973. *Religion, Altered States of Consciousness and Social Change*. Columbus: Ohio State University Press.

Boyle, R. 1685. *An Essay of the Great Effects of Even Languid and Unheeded Motion.* London: M. Flescher.

Bragaglia, A.G. 1949. 'La tarantella', *Ricreazione,* I: 36–55.

————. 1950. *Danze popolari italiane.* Rome: ENAL.

Brecht, B. 1964. *Schriften zum Theater.* Weimar: BD.V. Berlin.

Bronzini, G. 1976. 'Salento: aspetti geographici, ambientali e demologici', *Testi e temi di storia delle tradizioni popolari,* 5: 120–52.

Brook, P. 1993. *There Are No Secrets: Thoughts on Acting and Theatre.* London: Methuen.

————. 1998. *Threads of Time: A Memoir.* London: Methuen.

Brunetto, W. 1995. 'La Raccolta 24 degli Archivi di Etnomusicologia dell'Accademia Nazionale di Santa Cecilia', *EM Annuario degli Archivi di Etnomusicologia dell'Accademia Nazionale di Santa Cecilia,* III: 115–87.

Bruno, V. 1999. 'E al Malè turisti in delirio per la pizzica', *Leccesera,* 13–14 August: 5.

Buckland, T. (ed.) 1999. *Dance in the Field: Theory, Methods and Issues in Dance Ethnography.* New York: St Martin's Press.

————. 2006. *Dancing from Past to Present: Nation, Culture, Identities.* Madison: University of Wisconsin Press.

Burney, C. 1771. *The Present State of Music in France and Italy.* London: Becket.

Campelli, A. 1878. 'Sopra un caso di tarantolismo felicemente curato', *Morgagni,* 20: 538–43.

Caggia, D. 1984. 'Il ragno, la donna e il diavolo', *L'Immaginale: Rassegna di psicologia,* 3: 163–74.

Caputo, N. 1741. *De tarantulae anatome et morsu.* Lecce: Viverito.

Carducci, L. 1993. *Storia del Salento. La Terra d'Otranto dalle origini ai primi del cinquecento. Società, religione, economia, cultura.* Galatina: Congedo.

Carignani, B. 2004. *Una malattia culturale: la possessione rituale. Aspetti psicosociali e psicopatalogici del tarantismo.* Mesagne: Giordano.

Carlson, E. and M. Simpson. 1971. 'Tarantism or Hysteria: an American Case of 1801', *Journal of the History of Medicine and Allied Sciences,* 26: 293–302.

Carusi, G. 1848. 'Delle tarantole e del tarantismo', *Resoconti dell'accademia medico-chirurgica napoletana,* 175, II: 35.

Cassin, E. 1962. 'Ernesto De Martino, La terra del rimorso – contributo alla storia religiosa del Sud', *L'Homme,* II: 131–33.

Castiglione, M. and L. Stocchi. 1977. 'Il tarantismo oggi: proposte per una verifica', *La critica sociologica,* 11 (44): 43–69.

Chambers, E. 1999. *Native Tours: The Anthropology of Travel and Tourism.* Long Grove: Waveland Press.

Chernoff, J. 1981. *African Rhythm and African Sensibilities: Aesthetics and Social Action in African Musical Idioms.* Chicago: University of Chicago Press.

Chiaia, L. [1887] 1983. *Pregiudizi pugliesi. Tarantolismo, malefizio, i serpi di San Paolo, roba spicciola.* Bologna: Forni.

Chiriatti, L. 1995. *Morso d'amore. Viaggio nel tarantismo salentino.* Lecce: Capone.

————. 1996. 'Galatina e dintorni: appunti per un diario, 29 giugno 1995', *Pietre.* 4: 12.

———. 1997a. 'Appunti per un diario: Galatina 29 giugno 1997', *Pietre*. 6: 10.

———. (ed.). 1997b. *Tarantismo: un saggio di Giuseppe De Masi, 1874*. Tricase: Bleve.

———. 1998. *Opillopillopìopillopillopà: viaggio nella musica popolare salentina 1970–1998*. Calimera: Edizioni Aramirè.

Chiriatti, L. and G. Lapassade. 1985. 'Sessualità nella cultura salentina', *Pensionante dei Saraceni*, 1: 137–44.

Chiriatti, L. and A. Miscuglio. 2004. 'Osso, sottosso, sopraosso. Storie di santi e di coltelli. La danza spada a Torrepaduli', *Kurumuny*, 11.

Chiriatti, L. and I. Della Mea and C. Longhini. 2007. *Gianni Bosio – Clara Longhini, 1968. Una ricerca in Salento*. Martignano: Kurumuny.

Cid, F.X. 1787. *Tarantismo observado en España*. Madrid: Gonzalez.

Cirillo, D. 1771. 'Some Account of the Manna Tree and of the Tarantula', *Philosophical Transactions*, LX. London: Lockyer Davis, pp. 233–38.

Ciuffitelli, M. 2005a. 'A Familiar Voice I Never Heard: Discovering and Promoting Pizzica in the US', *Speaking Memory: Oral History, Oral Culture and Italians in America Conference, Los Angeles, 3–6 November 2005*. Los Angeles: American Italian Historical Association.

Cixous, H. and C. Clément (eds). 1986. *The Newly Born Woman*, trans. B. Wing. Minneapolis: Theory and History of Literature, 24.

Classen, C. (ed.). 2005. *The Book of Touch*. Oxford: Berg.

Cohen, A. 1993. *Masquerade Politics. Explorations in the Structure of Urban Cultural Movements*. Oxford: Berg.

Cohen, A.P. 1994. *Self-consciousness: An Alternative Anthropology of Identity*. London: Routledge.

———. 2000. 'Introduction. Discriminating Relations: Identity, Boundary and Authenticity', in A.P. Cohen (ed.), *Signifying Identities: Anthropological Perspectives on Boundaries and Contested Values*. London: Routledge, pp. 1–14.

Coleman, S. and J. Eade (eds). 2004. *Reframing Pilgrimage: Cultures in Motion*. London: Routledge.

Collu, R. 2005. *Personaggi ordinariamente straordinari del Salento: Riflessioni dialogiche su alcuni temi di ricerca antropologica*. Nardò: Besa.

Colonna, S., M. Cucurachi and M. Garofalo. 1997. 'Il "morso" del ragno al giovane contadino di Uggiano La Chiesa: avvelenamento da neurotossine di origine animale in un giovane agricoltore. Latrodectismo? Caso clinico', in L. Chiriatti (ed.), *Tarantismo*. Tricase: Bleve, pp. 45–54.

Colonna, S., M. Cucurachi and M. Garofalo. 2000. 'Avvelenamento da neurotossine di origine animale. Latrodectismo? Caso clinico', in G. Di Mitri (ed.), *Quarant'anni dopo De Martino*. Vol. 1. Nardò: Besa, pp. 171–79.

Comerford Peters, M. and C. Schreiner. 1990. *Flamenco: Gypsy Dance and Music from Andalusia*. New York: Amadeus.

Congedo, U. 1903. 'I Castriota Scanderbeg duchi di Galatina (1485–1561)', *Rivista storica salentina*, I: 152–83.

Connell, J. and C. Gibson. 2003. *Soundtracks: Popular Music, Identity and Place*. London: Routledge.

Convegno organizzato dal Comune di San Vito dei Normanni. 1999. *Rimorso. La tarantola tra scienza e letteratura*. Nardò: Besa.

Coppa, P. 1996. *Etnopsichiatria*. Milan: Il Saggiatore.

Costa A. and B. Costa. 1999. *La tarantella. Storia, aneddoti e curiosità del ballo popolare più famoso del mondo, espressione tipica del folklore napoletano*. Rome: Newton Compton.

Csordas, T. 1994. *Embodiment and Experience*. London: Cambridge University Press.

———. 1996. 'Imaginal Performance and Memory in Ritual Healing', in C. Laderman and M. Roseman (eds), *The Performance of Healing*. London: Routledge, pp. 91–113.

———. 2002. *Body/Meaning/Healing*. New York: Palgrave.

Csordas, T. and K. Kleinman. 1996. 'The Therapeutic Process', in C. Sargent and T. Johnson (eds), *Medical Anthropology*. Westport: Praeger, pp. 3–20.

Daniel, V. 1996. *Charred Lullabies: Chapters in an Anthropology of Violence*. Princeton: Princeton University Press.

Daniel, Y. 2005. *Dancing Wisdom: Embodied Knowledge in Haitian Vodou, Cuban Yoruba, and Bahian Candomble*. Urbana: University of Illinois Press.

Dauterman Maguire, E., H. Maguire and M. Duncan-Flowers. 1989. *Art and Holy Powers in the Early Christian House*. Urbana: University of Illinois Press.

Davis, J. 1969. 'Honour and Politics in Pisticci', *Proceedings of the Royal Anthropological Institute*, 69–82.

Del Giudice, L. 2003. 'Healing the Spider's Bite: "Ballad Therapy" and Tarantismo', in T. McKean (ed.), *The Flowering Thorn: International Ballad Studies*. Logan: Utah State University Press, pp. 23–33.

———. 2005. 'The Folk Music Revival and the Culture of *Tarantismo* in the Salento', in L. Del Giudice and N. van Deusen (eds), *Performing Ecstasies*. Ottawa: Institute of Mediaeval Music, pp. 217–72.

Del Giudice, L. and N. van Deusen (eds). 2005. *Performing Ecstasies: Music, Dance and Ritual in the Mediterranean*. Ottawa: Institute of Mediaeval Music.

Delle Donne, G. 1996. 'Nel Salento torna la tarantola', *La Gazzetta del Mezzogiorno*, 14 July: 9.

De Giorgi, P. 1999. *Tarantismo e rinascita*. Lecce: Argo.

———. 2002. *Pizzica-pizzica: la musica della rinascita*. Lecce: Pensa.

———. 2004. *L'estetica della tarantella: pizzica, mito e ritmo*. Galatina: Congedo.

———. 2005. *Pizzica e tarantismo: la carne del mito dall'etnomusicologia all'estetica musicale*. Galatina: Edit Santoro.

De Marra, G. 1362. *Sertum papale de venenis*. Bibl. Vaticana, Ms. Lat. Barberini 306.

De Martino, E. 1956. 'Crisi della presenza e reintegrazione religiosa', *Aut-aut*, 31: 17–38.

———. 1960. *Sud e magia*. Milan: Feltrinelli.

_____. 1961a. *La terra del rimorso: contributo a una storia religiosa del Sud.* Milan: Il Saggiatore.

_____. 1961b. 'Land der Gewissenspein', *Antaios*, 3(2): 105–24.

_____. 1966. *La terre du remords*, trans. C. Poncet. Paris: Gallimard.

_____. 1975. *Morte e pianto rituale: dal lamento funebre antico al pianto di Maria.* Turin: Einaudi.

_____. 1999. *La tierra del rimordimento*, trans. O.P. Rosario. Barcelona: Bellaterra.

_____. 2005. *The Land of Remorse: a Study of Southern Italian Tarantism*, trans. D.L. Zinn. London: Free Association Books.

De Masi, G. 1874. 'Sul tarantolismo: lettera ad un amico', *Gazzetta medica di Puglia*, 5.

De Raho, F. [1908] 1994. *Il tarantolismo nella superstizione e nella scienza.* Rome: Sensibili alle foglie.

Desjarlais, R. 1992. *Body and Emotion: The Aesthetics of Illness and Healing in the Nepal Himalayas.* Philadelphia: University of Pennsylvania Press.

_____. 1996. 'Presence', in C. Laderman and M. Roseman (eds). *The Performance of Healing.* London: Routledge, pp. 143–64.

_____. 2003. *Sensory Biographies: Lives and Deaths Among Nepal's Yolmo Buddhists.* Berkeley: University of California Press.

Devish, R. 1993. *Weaving the Threads of Life: the Khita Gyn-Eco-Logical Healing Cult Among the Yaka.* Chicago: Chicago University Press.

Di Ciaula, T. 2001. *Il dio delle tarantate.* Castelfranco: Libro Press.

Dijkstra, B. 1996. *Evil Sisters: The Threat of Female Sexuality in Twentieth-Century Culture.* New York: Henry Holt.

Dils, A. and A. Cooper Albright (eds). 2001. *Moving History/Dancing Cultures: A Dance History Reader.* Middletown: Wesleyan University Press.

Di Lecce, G. 1992. 'La danza scherma salentina', *Lares*, LVIII,1: 33–45.

_____. 1994. *La danza della piccola taranta. Cronache da Galatina: 1908–1993. A memoria d'uomo.* Rome: Sensibili alle foglie.

_____. 1998. 'Danza popolare e animazione sociale', *Quaderni del Dipartimento di Scienze dei Sistemi Sociali e della Comunicazione*, 4: 161–86.

_____. 2001a. 'Cuore e ritmo: la comunicazione del duemila', *Quotidiano di Lecce.* 219: 1–7.

_____. 2001b. *Tretarante: taranta/pizzica/scherma. Le tarantelle-pizziche del Salento.* Nardò: Besa.

Di Mitri, G. 1995. 'La terra del rimosso: tarantismo e medicina nell'area galatinese in età moderna', *Bollettino storico di Terra d'Otranto*, 5: 221–29.

_____. 1996. 'Le radici orfiche e l'innesto paolino sul tronco del tarantismo. Ipotesi e indizi per un'archeologia del sapere', in M. Paone (ed.), *Scritti di storia pugliese in onore di Feliciano Argentina*, Vol. 1. Galatina: Congedo, pp. 11–28.

_____. (ed.). 2000. *Quarant'anni dopo De Martino. Atti del convegno internazionale di studi sul tarantismo*, Vols I and II. Nardò: Besa.

_____. 2001. 'Un patrimonio da salvare', *Quotidiano di Lecce*, 226: 1, 6.

————. 2006. *Storia biomedica del tarantismo nel XVIII secolo.* Florence: Leo S. Olschki.

Doménech y Amaya, P. [1792] 1998. *Indagine su un uomo morso dalla tarantola*, trans. L. Apa. Palermo: Sellerio.

Douglas, M. 1966. *Purity and Danger: An Analysis of Concepts of Pollution and Taboo.* London: Routledge.

Downey, G. 2005. *Learning Capoeira: Lessons in Cunning from an Afro-Brazilian Art.* Oxford: Oxford University Press.

Driessen, H. 2002. 'People, Boundaries and the Anthropologist's Mediterranean', *Anthropological Journal on European Cultures*, 10: 11–24.

Dubisch, J. and M. Winkelman. 2005. *Pilgrimage and Healing.* Tucson: University of Arizona Press.

Durante, D. 1999. 'Pizzica e techno pizzica', in V. Ampolo and G. Zappatore (eds), *Musica, droga e transe.* Rome: Sensibili alle foglie, pp. 167–90.

————. 2005. *Spartito (io resto qui): storie e canzoni della musica popolare salentina.* Lecce: Salento Altra Musica.

Durante, R. 1998. 'Se vive la musica popolare resta accesa la memoria del passato', *Quotidiano di Lecce*, 173: 10.

Epifani, M. 1998. *Ematoritmi: La donna nella tradizione e nei canti dell'area messapica.* Lecce: Editore Manni.

Fabris, D. 2005. 'Il business Notte della Taranta, non spacciamolo per nobile', *La Repubblica*, 29 July: X.

Farnell, B. 1999. 'Moving Bodies, Acting Selves', *Annual Review of Anthropology*, 28: 341–73.

Feld, S. 1990. *Sound and Sentiment: Birds, Weeping, Poetics, and Song in Kaluli Expression.* Philadelphia: University of Pennsylvania Press.

————. 2000. 'A Sweet Lullaby for World Music', *Public Culture*, 12(1): 145–71.

Ferdinando, E. 1621. *Centum historiae seu observationes et casus medici.* Venice: Apud T. Baglionum.

Ferrari de Nigris, D. (ed.). 1997. *Musica, rito e aspetti terapeutici nella cultura mediterranea.* Genoa: Erga Edizioni.

Filipucci, P. 1996. 'Anthropological Perspectives on Culture in Italy', in D. Forgacs (ed.), *Italian Cultural Studies.* Oxford: Oxford University Press, pp. 52–71.

Forgacs, D. 1996. *Italian Cultural Studies.* Oxford: Oxford University Press.

Franco, O. and S. Zuffi. 1996. *Musica maga: teoresi e storia della meloterapia dei poteri terapeutici e fascinatori della musica.* Genoa: Erga Edizioni.

Friedman, R. 1978. '"If You Don't Play Good They Take the Drum Away": Performance, Communication and Acts in Guagnanco', in C. Card, J. Hasse, R. Singer and R. Stone (eds), *Discourse in Ethnomusicology: Essays in Honor of George List.* Bloomington: Indiana University Press, pp. 209–24.

Fumarola, P. 1998. 'Produzione e riscatto con la musica popolare', *Quotidiano di Lecce*, 174: IV.

Gala, G. 2002a. '"La *pizzica* ce l'ho nel sangue": Riflessioni a margine sul ballo tradizionale e sulla nuova pizzicomania del Salento', in S. Torsello and V. Santoro (eds), *Il ritmo meridiano.* Lecce, Aramirè, pp. 109–53.

──── . 2002b. 'Mitificazioni coreo-musicali e nuovi linguaggi corporei', in A. Lamanna (ed.), *Ragnatele*. Rome: Adnkronos, pp. 40–55.

Galanti, B. 1950. *Dances of Italy*. London: Max Parrish.

Gallini, C. 1967. *I rituali dell'argia*. Padua: Cedam.

──── . 1982. 'Ernesto De Martino: Vorläufer, Lebenswerk und Nachfolger', in H. Nixdorf and T. Hauschild (eds), *Europäische Ethnologie*. Berlin: Dietrich Raimer, pp. 221–41.

──── . 1988 *La ballerina variopinta: una festa di guarigione in Sardegna*. Naples: Liguori.

Gallini, C. and F. Faeta, (eds). 1999. *I viaggi nel Sud di Ernesto De Martino*. Turin: Bollati Boringhieri.

Gentilcore, D. 1992. *From Bishop to Witch: The System of the Sacred in Early Modern Terra d'Otranto*. Manchester: Manchester University Press.

──── . 1998. *Healers and Healing in Early Modern Italy*. Manchester: Manchester University Press.

──── . 2000. 'Ritualised Illness and Music Therapy: Views of Tarantism in the Kingdom of Naples', in P. Horden (ed.), *Music as Medicine*. Aldershot: Ashgate, pp. 255–72.

Geurtz, K. 2002. *Culture and the Senses: Bodily Ways of Knowing in an African Community*. Berkeley: University of California Press.

Giannuzzi, C. 1996. *Il dio che danza*. Maglie: Erreci Edizioni.

Gilbert, S. 1986. 'Introduction: a Tarantella of Theory', in H. Cixous and C. Clément (eds), *The Newly Born Woman*, trans. B. Wing. Minneapolis: Theory and History of Literature, 24, pp. ix–xviii.

Gingrich, A. 2004. 'Conceptualising Identities: Anthropological Alternatives to Essentialising Difference and Moralizing about Othering', in G. Baumann and A. Gingrich (eds), *Grammars of Identity/Alterity: A Structural Approach*. Oxford: Berghahn, pp. 3–17.

Ginsborg, P. 1990. *A History of Contemporary Italy: Society and Politics, 1943–1988*. Harmondsworth: Penguin.

Giordano, C. 1992. *Die Betrogenen der Geschichte: Überlagerungsmentalität und Überlagerungsrationalität in mediterranen Gesellschaften*. Frankfurt am Main: Campus.

──── . 2002. 'Mediterranean Honour Reconsidered', *Anthropological Journal on European Cultures*, 10: 39–58.

Giordano, E. 1957. 'Una particolare forma di psicosi collettiva: il tarantulismo', *Neuropsichiatria*, XIII(I): 43–76.

Goddard, V. 1987. 'Honour and Shame: the Control of Women's Sexuality and Group Identity in Naples', in P. Caplan (ed.), *The Cultural Construction of Sexuality*. London: Tavistock, pp. 166–93.

──── . 1996. *Gender, Family and Work in Naples*. Oxford: Berg.

Goddard, V., J. Llobera, and C. Shore. 1996. 'From the Mediterranean to Europe: Honour, Kinship and Gender', in V. Goddard, J. Llobera and C. Shore (eds), *The Anthropology of Europe*. Oxford: Berg, pp. 1–40.

Gouk, P. (ed.). 2000. *Musical Healing in Cultural Contexts*. Aldershot: Ashgate.

Gramsci, A. 1965. *Lettere dal carcere*. Turin: Einaudi.

————. 1985. *Selections from Cultural Writings*. London: Lawrence and Wishart.

Graziosi, P. 1996. *The Prehistoric Paintings of the Porto Badisco Cave*. Pisa: Edizioni ETS.

Grenier L. and J. Guilbault. 1990. '"Authority" Revisited: the "Other" in Anthropology and Popular Music Studies', *Ethnomusicology*, 34(3): 381–97.

Gribaudi, G. 1996. 'Images of the South', in D. Forgacs (ed.), *Italian Cultural Studies*. Oxford: Oxford University Press, pp. 72–87.

Grotowski, J. 1976. *Towards a Poor Theatre*. London: Methuen.

Guerra-Lisi, S. 1987. *Il metodo della globalità dei linguaggi: educazione motoria al suono e all'immagine*. Rome: Edizioni Borla.

Gupta, A. and J. Ferguson (eds). 1997. *Culture, Power, Place: Explorations in Critical Anthropology*. Durham: Duke University Press.

Guss, D. 2000. *The Festive State: Race, Ethnicity and Nationalism as Cultural Performance*. Berkeley: University of California Press.

Hagedorn, K. 2001. *Divine Utterances: The Performance of Afro-Cuban Santería*. Washington, DC: Smithsonian Institution Press.

Hall, E. 1983. *The Dance of Life: the Other Dimension of Time*. New York: Anchor Books.

Hamayon, R. 1995. 'Are "Trance," "Ecstasy" and Similar Concepts Appropriate in the Study of Shamanism?' in T. Kim and M. Hoppál (eds), *Shamanism in Performing Arts*. Budapest: Akadémiai Kiadò, pp. 17–34.

Hanna, J. 1979. *To Dance is Human: A Theory of Nonverbal Communication*. Chicago: Chicago University Press.

Harris, R. 2000. *Body and Spirit in the Secular Age*. London: Penguin Books.

Hecker, J. 1865. *Die Großen Volkskrankheiten des Mittelalters*. Berlin: Enslin.

Helman, C. 1984. *Culture, Health and Illness*. Bristol: Wright.

Herzfeld, M. 1987. *Anthropology Through the Looking-Glass: Critical Ethnography in the Margins of Europe*. Cambridge: Cambridge University Press.

Hobsbawn, E. 1983. 'Introduction', in E. Hobsbawm and T. Ranger (eds), *The Invention of Tradition*. Cambridge: Cambridge University Press, pp. 1–14.

Hobsbawm, E. and T. Ranger (eds). 1983. *The Invention of Tradition*. Cambridge: Cambridge University Press.

Horden, P. (ed.). 2000. *Music as Medicine: the History of Music Therapy since Antiquity*. Aldershot: Ashgate.

————. 2003. 'Continuità e discontinuità nella storia della terapia musicale nel Mediterraneo', in M. Agamennone and G. Di Mitri (eds), *L'eredità di Diego Carpitella: etnomusicologia, antropologia e ricerca storica nel Salento e nell'area mediterranea*. Nardò: Besa, pp. 187–97.

Howes, D. (ed.). 1992. *The Varieties of Sensory Experience*. Toronto: University of Toronto Press.

————. 2004. *Empire of the Senses: the Sensual Culture Reader*. Oxford: Berg.

Hsu, E. 2005. 'Acute Pain Infliction as Therapy', *Etnofoor*, 18(1): 78–95.

Hsu, E. and C. Low. (eds). 2007. 'Wind, Life and Health: Anthropological Perspectives', *JRAI Special Volume*.

Imbriani, E. 2001. 'Se la taranta non ha paura di rinnovarsi', *Quotidiano di Lecce*, 218: 1–9.

Imbriani, E. and P. Fumarola (eds). 2007. *Danze di corteggiamento e di sfida nel mondo globalizzato*. Nardò: Besa.

Inchingolo, R. 2003. *Luigi Stifani e la pizzica tarantata*. Nardò: Besa.

Inda, J. and R. Rosaldo (eds). 2002. *The Anthropology of Globalization: A Reader*. Oxford: Blackwell.

Indennitate, G. 2005. 'Taranta e Treccani. Una Puglia "enciclopedica"', *Gazzetta del Mezzogiorno*, 26 August: 20.

———. 2006. 'Cina? Missione possibile', *Gazzetta del Mezzogiorno*, 11 May: Lecce 5.

Inguscio, E. 2007. *La pizzica scherma di Torrepaduli: San Rocco, la festa, il mito, il santuario*. Copertino: Lupo Editore.

Jennings, S. (ed.). 1994. *The Handbook of Dramatherapy*. London: Routledge.

———. 1995. *Theatre, Ritual and Transformation: the Senoi Temiars*. London: Routledge.

Jervis, G. 1961. 'Considerazioni neuropsichiatriche sul tarantismo', in E. De Martino, *La terra del rimorso*, Appendix I. Milan: Il Saggiatore, pp. 287–306.

———. 1962. 'Il tarantolismo pugliese', *Il lavoro neuropsichiatrico*, 16: 297–360.

Jones, D. (ed.). 2002. *Combat, Ritual and Performance: Anthropology of the Martial Arts*. Westport: Praeger.

Jurlaro, R. 1980. 'Il fenomeno del tarantolismo in Puglia', *Rassegna salentina*. 5: 55–66.

Kaeppler, A. 2000. 'Dance Ethnology and the Anthropology of Dance', *Dance Research Journal*, 32(1): 116–25.

Katner, W. 1952. 'Musik und Medizin im Zeitalter des Barock', *Wissenschaftliche Zeitschrift der Karl Marx Universität*, 7/8: 477–508.

———. 1956. 'Das Rätsel des Tarantismus: eine Ätiologie der italienischen Tanzkrankheit', *Nova acta leopoldina*, 18(124): 1–115.

Kinsley, D. 1995. *The Goddesses' Mirror: Visions of the Divine from East to West*. Delhi: Sri Satguru Publications.

Kircher, A. 1641/1654. *Magnes sive de arte magnetica*. Rome: Tipographia Ludovici Grignani.

———. 1673. *Phonurgia nova*. Campidoniae: Rudolphum Dreherr.

Kirtsoglou, E. and D. Theodossopoulos, 2004. 'They are Taking our Culture Away: Tourism and Culture Commodification in the Garifuna Community of Roatan', *Critique of Anthropology*, 24(2): 135–57.

Kleinman, A. 1980. *Patients and Healers in the Context of Culture*. Berkeley: University of California Press.

Kobert, R. 1901. *Beiträge zur Kenntnis der Giftspinnen*. Stuttgart: Enke.

Kümmel, W. 1977. *Musik und Medizin: Ihre Wechselbeziehungen in Theorie und Praxis von 800 bis 1800*. Munich: Karl Alber Freiburg.

Laderman, C. 1981. 'Symbolic and Empirical Reality: a New Approach to the Analysis of Food Avoidances', *American Ethnologist*, 8(3): 468–93.

———. 1991. *Taming the Wind of Desire: Psychology, Medicine and Aesthetics in Malay Shamanistic Performance*. Berkeley: University of California Press.

———. 1996. 'The Poetics of Healing in Malay Shamanistic Performances', in C. Laderman and M. Roseman (eds), *The Performance of Healing*. London: Routledge, pp. 115–41.

Laderman, C. and M. Roseman (eds). 1996. *The Performance of Healing*. London: Routledge.

Lamanna, A. (ed.). 2002. *Ragnatele: tarantismo, danza, musica e nuove identità nel Sud d'Italia*. Rome: Adnkronos.

Lanternari, V. 1995. 'Tarantismo: dal medico neopositivista all'antropologo, alla etnopsichiatria di oggi', *Storia, antropologia e scienze del linguaggio*, 3: 67–92.

———. 2000. 'Tarantismo: vecchie teorie, saperi nuovi', in G. Di Mitri (ed.), *Quarant'anni dopo De Martino*, Vol. II. Nardò: Besa, pp. 119–34.

Lapassade, G. 1994. *Intervista sul tarantismo*. Maglie: Madonna Oriente.

———. 1996a. *Stati modificati e transe*. Rome: Sensibili alle foglie.

———. 1996b. *Transe e dissociazione*. Rome: Sensibili alle foglie.

———. 1997. *Les Rites de possession*. Paris: Anthropos.

———. 2001. *Dal candomblè al tarantismo*. Rome: Sensibili alle foglie.

Lazzari, F. 1972. *Esperienze religiose e psicoanalisi*. Naples: Guida Editori.

León Sanz, P. 2000. 'Medical Theories of Tarantism in Eighteenth-century Spain', in P. Horden (ed.), *Music as Medicine*. Aldershot: Ashgate, pp. 273–92.

———. 2008. *La tarantola spagnola: empirismo e tradizione nel XVIII secolo*. Nardò: Besa

Lewis, I. 1971. *Ecstatic Religion: an Anthropological Study of Spirit Possession and Shamanism*. Harmondsworth: Penguin.

———. 1991. 'The Spider and the Pangolin', *Man*, 26(3): 513–25.

Ligori, V., L. Manni and M. Cazzato. 2001. *Sulle tracce di San Paolo. Verità storiche e invenzioni tarantologiche*. Galatina: Torgraf.

Littlewood, R. 1990. 'From Categories to Contexts: a Decade of the "New Cross-cultural Psychiatry"', *British Journal of Psychiatry*. 156: 308–27.

Livingston, T. 1999. 'Music Revivals: Towards a General Theory', *Ethnomusicology*, 43(1): 66–85.

Lock, M. 1993. 'Cultivating the Body: Anthropology and Epistemologies of Bodily Practice and Knowledge', *Annual Review of Anthropology*, 22: 133–55.

Lock, M. and N. Scheper-Hughes. 1996. 'A Critical-interpretive Approach in Medical Anthropology: Rituals and Routines of Discipline and Dissent', in C. Sargent and T. Johnson (eds), *Medical Anthropology*. Westport: Praeger, pp. 41–70.

Lombardi Satriani, R. 1951. *Credenze popolari calabresi*. Naples: De Simone.

Lorenzetti, R. 1982. 'Ernesto De Martino e le tarantate del Salento', *Sallentum*, 1: 9–34.

Lowell Lewis, J. 1992. *Ring of Liberation: Deceptive Discourse in Brazilian Capoeira*. Chicago: Chicago University Press.

Lüdtke, K. 2000a. 'Tarantism in Contemporary Italy: the Tarantula's Dance Reviewed and Revived', in P. Horden (ed.), *Music as Medicine*. Aldershot: Ashgate, pp. 293–312.

———. 2000b. 'Theatre and Therapy: the Tarantula's Dance in Salento, Italy'. DPhil Thesis. Oxford University.

———. 2002. 'Le arti, l'habitat e il benessere nell'ottica prospettica dell'antropologia medica: il tarantismo nel Salento', in *Medicina e Storia*, 3: 119–28.

———. 2003. 'Dal rito della taranta alla musicoterapia odierna: note fra storia e antropologia', in M. Agamennone and G. Di Mitri (eds), *L'eredità di Diego Carpitella*. Nardò: Besa, pp. 147–61.

———. 2005a. 'Dancing Towards Well-Being: Reflections on the *Pizzica* in the Contemporary Salento, Italy', in L. Del Giudice and N. van Deusen (eds), *Performing Ecstasies*. Ottawa: Institute of Mediaeval Music, pp. 37–53.

———. 2005b. '"Non si sopravviverebbe senza un'identità": identificazione e trasformazione', *Melissi*, 10/11: 129–31.

Maalouf, A. 2000. *On Identity*. London: Harvill.

MacCannell, D. 1999. *The Tourist*. New York: Schocken.

MacKinlay, E., D. Collins and S. Owens (eds). 2005. *Aesthetics and Experience in Music Performance*. Cambridge: Cambridge Scholars Press.

Maggiorelli, S. 1996. 'Dalla tarantola alla tecno', *Liberazione*, 4 December: 25.

Malaterra, G. 1724. 'Historia sicula, De rebus gestis Rogerii Calabriae et Siciliae comitis', II.36. *Rerum Italicarum Scriptores V*. Milan: L.A. Muratori.

Marino, N. (ed.). 2007. *Mordi e fuggi. 16 racconti per evadere dalla taranta*. Lecce: Manni.

Maruccio, V. 1999. 'La febbre della notte nei tempi della musica: la "pizzica" dall'aia in discoteca', *Quotidiano di Lecce*, XXI(189): 4–5.

———. 2005. 'Il ragno "morde" anche il turismo. Boom nel Salento', *Quotidiano di Lecce*, 26 August: 11.

Massari, A. 1998. *Edoardo*. Milan: Edizioni D'Ars.

Mathews, G. and C. Izquierdo. 2008. *Pursuits of Happiness: Well-being in Anthropological Perspective*. Oxford: Berghahn.

Mauss, M. 1979. *Sociology and Psychology*. London: Routledge.

McNeill, W. 1995. *Keeping Together in Time: Dance and Drill in Human History*. Cambridge: Harvard University Press.

Meis, A. 2006. 'Se ci danno 20mila € espitiamo pure noi l'Orchestra', *Nuovo Quotidiano di Puglia*, 12 May: 12.

Melchioni, E. 1999. *Zingari, San Rocco, pizzica-scherma: per una storia socio-culturale dei rom nel mezzogiorno*. Lecce: Novaracne.

Merriam, A. 1964. *The Anthropology of Music*. Evanston: Northwestern University Press.

Metafune, A. 2002. 'Era molto meglio prima. Anzi no', *Piazza del Popolo*, August: 7.

Mina, G. 1997. 'Se la taranta è sorda. Un aspetto inconsueto del tarantismo pugliese', in D. Ferrari De Nigris (ed.), *Musica, rito e aspetti terapeutici nella cultura mediterranea*. Genoa: Erga, pp. 119–26.

———. 2000. *Il morso della differenza. Antologia del dibattito sul tarantismo fra il XIV e il XVI secolo*. Nardò, Besa.

Mina, G. and S. Torsello (eds). 2006. *La tela infinita: bibliografia degli studi sul tarantismo mediterraneo 1945–2006*. Nardò: Besa.

Mingozzi. G. 2002. *La taranta*. Nardò: Besa.

Mitchell, S. 1998. 'The Theatre of Self-expression: Seven Approaches to an Interactional Ritual Theatre Form', *Dramatherapy*, 20(1): 3–10.

Monaco, D. 2006. *La scherma salentina ... a memoria d'uomo*. Lecce. Aramirè.

Montinaro, B. 1976. *Salento povero*. Ravenna: Longo.

———. 1996. *San Paolo dei serpenti. Analisi di una tradizione*. Palermo: Sellerio.

———. 2007. *Danzare col ragno. Musica e letteratura sul tarantismo dal XV al XX secolo*. Lecce: Argo.

Moore, H. 1994. 'Understanding Sex and Gender', in T. Ingold (ed.), *Companion Encyclopedia of Anthropology*. London: Routledge, pp. 813–30.

Moore, R. 2003. 'Review: Divine Utterances: the Performance of Afro-Cuban Santería by Katherine Hagedorn', *Latin American Music Review*, 24(1): 153–55.

Mora, G. 1963. 'An Historical and Sociopsychiatric Appraisal of Tarantism and its Importance in the Tradition of Psychotherapy of Mental Disorders', *Bulletin of the History of Medicine*, 37: 417–39.

Morley, D. and K. Robins, 1995. *Spaces of Identity: Global Media, Electronic Landscapes and Cultural Boundaries*. London: Routledge.

Morris, B. 1994. *Anthropology of the Self: the Individual in Cultural Perspective*. London: Pluto Press.

Myers, H. 1984. 'Ethnomusicology', in *New Grove Dictionary of American Music*. London: Macmillan.

Nacci, A. (ed.). 2001. *Tarantismo e neotarantismo. Musica, danza, transe. Bisogni di oggi, bisogni di sempre*. Nardò: Besa.

———. 2004. *Neotarantismo*. Viterbo: Nuovi Equilibri.

Naselli, C. 1951. 'L'etimologia di "tarantella"', *Archivio storico pugliese*, IV: 218–27.

Negro, M. and C. Sergio. 2000. 'La musica popolare nella reinterpretazione della nuova generazione'. Tesina di antropologia culturale. Università di Lecce.

Ness, S. 1992. *Body, Movement and Culture: Kinesthetic and Visual Symbolism in a Philippine Community*. Philadelphia: University of Pennsylvania Press.

Nettl, B. 1983. *The Study of Ethnomusicology: Twenty-nine Issues and Concepts*. Urbana: University of Illinois Press.

Nichter, M. and M. Lock (eds). 2002. *New Horizons in Medical Anthropology: Essays in Honour of Charles Lesile*. London: Routledge.

Nocera, M. 1994. 'Nella cappella di San Paolo, suonando il tamburo rullante', in G. Di Lecce (ed.), *La danza della piccola taranta*. Rome: Sensibili alle foglie, pp. 178–86.

———. 2005. *Il morso del ragno: alle origini del tarantismo*. Lecce: Capone.

Ovid. 1957. *Metamorphoses*. London: Calder.

Pandolfi, M. 1990. 'Boundaries Inside the Body: Women's Suffering in Southern Peasant Italy', *Culture, Medicine and Psychiatry*, 14: 255–73.

Panico, F. 1983. *Il vestito bianco*. Milan: Garbagnate Milanese.

Parkin, D. (ed.). 1996. *The Politics of Performance*. Oxford: Berghahn.

Patruno, F. 2003. 'Le categorie antropologiche nella pizzica (mazzate pesanti)', retrieved on 8 February 2008 from www.pizzicata.it discussion forum.

Pellegrino, G. 1995. 'Passione e resurrezione del tamburello', *Pietre*, 0: 15.

————. 2002. 'Tra notti e festival, attenti a non soffocare la festa in onore di San Rocco', *Nuovo Quotidiano di Puglia*, 5 October: VII.

Peristiany, J. 1965. *Honour and Shame: the Values of Mediterranean Society*. Nature of Human Society Series. London: Weidenfeld and Nicolson.

Peterson Royce, A. 1977. *The Anthropology of Dance*. Bloomington: Indiana University Press.

————. 2004. *Anthropology of the Performing Arts: Artistry, Virtuosity and Interpretation in a Cross-cultural Perspective*. Lanham: Altamira Press.

Pinna, F. 2002. *I viaggi nel Sud di Ernesto De Martino*. Turin: Bollati Boringhieri.

Pitré, G. [1894] 1949. *Medicina popolare siciliana*. Florence: Barbera.

Pizza, G. 2002a. 'Lettera a Sergio Torsello e Vincenzo Santoro sopra il tarantismo, l'antropologia e le politiche della cultura', in S. Torsello and V. Santoro (eds), *Il ritmo meridiano*. Lecce: Aramirè, pp. 43–63.

————. 2002b. 'Retoriche del tarantismo e politiche culturali', in A. Lamanna (ed.), *Ragnatele*. Rome: Adnkronos, pp. 68–78.

Portulano Scoditti, M. (ed). 1999. *Epifanio Ferdinando. Medico, storico, filosofo. Mesagne 1569–1638. La vita e brani scelti dalle sue centum historiae*. Nardò: Besa.

Post, J. (ed.). 2006. *Ethnomusicology: a Contemporary Reader*. London: Routledge.

Presicce, C. 1999. 'La nuova forza della "taranta" nelle immagini di Bevilacqua', *Quotidiano di Lecce*, 30 June: 11.

————. 2005. 'Anche i cinesi ballano la pizzica', *Nuovo Quotidiano di Puglia*, 7 August: 23.

————. 2006. 'La Taranta ha gli occhi a mandorla', *Nuovo Quotidiano di Puglia*, 3 May: 25.

Probo, L. 1996. 'Santu Roccu meu, ci me vardi tie, l'otri li consu ieu'. *Pietre. Speciale San Rocco*, I(6): 2.

Quarta, D. 2007a. *La Notte della Taranta: breve storia per testi e immagini dei dieci anni che hanno 'rivoluzionato' la musica popolare salentina*. Lecce: Guitar.

————. 2007b. 'La pizzica si riscopre multietnica e Pagani incontra i canti di Puglia', in *quiSalento*, 15 July – 5 August, 7(8): 77.

Raheja, G. and A. Gold. (eds). 1994. *Listen to the Heron's Words: Reimagining Gender and Kinship in North India*. Berkeley: University of California Press.

Raheli, R. 1998. 'E così ritornammo a parlare di notti e di tarante', *Quotidiano di Lecce*, 168: XVI.

————. 2005. 'Pizzica Tarantata: Reflections of a Violin Player', in L. Del Giudice and N. van Deusen (eds), *Performing Ecstasies*. Ottawa: Institute of Mediaeval Music, pp. 125–28.

Raheli, R., V. Santoro and S. Torsello (eds). 2004. *Aloisi, Uccio. I colori della terra: canti e racconti di un musicista popolare*. Lecce: Aramirè.

Rapport, N. 2003. *I Am Dynamite: An Alternative Anthropology of Power*. London: Routledge.

Rapport, N. and V. Amit. 2002. *The Trouble with Community: Anthropological Reflections on Movement, Identity and Collectivity*. London: Pluto Press.

Reed, S. 1998. 'The Politics and Poetics of Dance', *Annual Review of Anthropology.* 27: 503–32.

Risso, M. and W. Böker. 1964. *Verhexungswahn: Ein Beitrag zum Verständnis von Wahnerkrankungen süditalienischer Arbeiter in der Schweiz.* Basle: S. Karger.

Rivera, A. 1996. 'Tarantismo. Può tornare? Dopo il recente caso in Salento', *La Gazzetta del Mezzogiorno*, 20 July: 17.

Rohlfs, G. 1956–1961. *Vocabolario dei dialetti salentini (Terra d'Otranto)*, 3 Vols. Munich: Verlag der Bayrischen Akademie der Wissenschaften.

Romanazzi, A. 2006. *Il ritorno del dio che balla: culti e riti del tarantolismo in Italia.* Rome: Venexia.

Romano, M. 2006. 'Triciu: dalla pizzica al punk-dub-tarantolato', *quiSalento*, April: 52.

Roseman, M. 1993. *Healing Sounds from the Malaysian Rainforest: Temiar Music and Medicine.* Berkeley: University of California Press.

———. 1996. 'Pure Products Go Crazy: Rainforest Healing in a Nation State', in C. Laderman and M. Roseman (eds). *The Performance of Healing.* London: Routledge, pp. 233–69.

———. 2002. 'Making Sense out of Modernity', in M. Nichter and M. Lock (eds), *New Horizons in Medical Anthropology: Essays in Honour of Charles Lesile.* London: Routledge, pp. 111–40.

Rossi, A. 1970. *Lettere da una tarantata.* Bari: De Donato.

———. 1991. *E il mondo si fece giallo. Il tarantismo in Campania.* Vibo Valentia: Qualecultura/Jaca Book.

Rouget, G. 1986. *Music and Trance: a Theory of the Relations Between Music and Possession*, trans. B. Biebuyck. Chicago: Chicago University Press.

Rowling, J.K. 1998. *Harry Potter and the Chamber of Secrets.* London: Bloomsbury.

Russell, J. 1979. 'Tarantism', *Medical History*, 23: 404–25.

Sadie, S. (ed.). 1980. *New Grove Dictionary of Music and Musicians.* Oxford: Oxford University Press.

Salvatore, G. 1989. *Isole sonanti: scenari archetipici della musica del mediterraneo*, Vol. 1. Rome: Il Ventaglio.

———. 2000. 'Oltre De Martino. Per una rifondazione degli studi sul tarantismo', in G. Di Mitri (ed.), *Quarant'anni dopo De Martino. Atti del convegno internazionale di studi sul tarantismo*, Vol. I. Nardò: Besa, pp. 11–49.

Sant Cassia, P. 2000. 'Exoticizing Discoveries and Extraordinary Experiences: "Traditional" Music, Modernity and Nostalgia in Malta and Other Mediterranean Societies', *Ethnomusicology*, 44(2): 281–301.

Sante Ardoini. [1426] 1492. *Sertum papale de venenis.* Venetiis.

Santoro, L. 1982. 'Macare e tarante', *Quaderni di Teatro*, 18: 71–82.

———. 1987. 'Il Paese dove il ragno canta', *Hyphos*, 1: 62–70.

———. 2001. 'E se la taranta si vendicasse?' *Quotidiano di Lecce*, 217: 1–6.

Santoro, V. 2001. 'La pizzica piace così: perchè contaminarla?' *Quotidiano di Lecce*, 220: 1–7.

———. 2005a. 'Il "movimento della pizzica" e la politica delle istituzioni locali', *Melissi*, 10/11: 92–96.

———. 2005b. 'Una fondazione ad hoc per la Notte della Taranta. Il movimento della pizzica solleva l'esigenza di una legge regionale per valorizzare la musica popolare pugliese', *La Repubblica*, 21 July.

Santoro, V. and S. Torsello (eds). 2002. *Il ritmo meridiano. La pizzica e le identità danzanti del Salento*. Lecce, Aramirè.

Sargent, C. and T. Johnson. 1996. *Medical Anthropology: Contemporary Theory and Method*. Westport: Praeger.

Saunders, G. 1984. 'Contemporary Italian Cultural Anthropology', *Annual Review of Anthropology*, 13: 447–66.

Savigliano, E. 1995. *Tango and the Political Economy of Passion: From Exoticism to Decolonization*. Boulder: Westview Press.

Sax, W. 2004. 'Healing Rituals: a Critical Performative Approach', *Anthropology of Medicine*, 11(3): 293–306.

Schechner, R. 1985. *Between Theatre and Anthropology*. Philadelphia: University of Pennsylvania Press.

———. 1988. *Performance Theory*. London: Routledge.

———. (ed). 2002. *Performance Studies: An Introduction*. London: Routledge.

Scheper-Hughes, N. and M. Lock. 1987. 'The Mindful Body: a Prolegomenon to Future Work in Medical Anthropology', *Medical Anthropological Quarterly*, New Series, 1(1): 6–32.

Schieffelin, E. 1996. 'On Failure and Performance: Throwing the Medium out of the Séance', in C. Laderman and M. Roseman (eds), *The Performance of Healing*. London: Routledge, pp. 59–89.

Schmeer, G. 2001. *Il panno rosso: dove si narra di un uomo pizzicato dalla tarantola*. Lecce: Capone.

Schneider, J. (ed). 1998. *Italy's 'Southern Question': Orientalism in One Country*. Oxford, New York: Berg.

Schneider, J. and P. Schneider. 1971. 'Of Vigilance and Virgins', *Ethnology*, 10: 1–24.

Schneider, M. 1948. *La danza de espadas y la tarantela. Ensayo musicológico, etnográfico y arqueológico sobre los ritos medicinales*. Barcelona: Instituto Español de Musicología.

Scholes, P. 1964. *Concise Oxford Dictionary of Music*. Oxford: Oxford University Press.

Schott-Billmann, F. 1994. *Quand la danse guérit*. Paris: Chiron.

Schullian, D. and M. Schoen (eds). 1948. *Music and Medicine*. New York: Henry Schuman.

Sechì, G. 1998. 'Le tarante pizzicano e ballano nel vuoto di cultura popolare', *Quotidiano di Lecce*. 174: XIV.

Seeger, A. 1987. *Why Suja Sing: the Anthropology of an Amazonian People*. Cambridge: Cambridge University Press.

Serao, F. 1742. *Della tarantola o sia falangio di Puglia*. Naples, pp. 95–96.

Sigerist, H. 1948. 'The Story of Tarantism', in D. Schullian and M. Schoen (eds), *Music and Medicine*. New York: Henry Schuman, pp. 96–116.

Silverman, S. 1968. 'Agricultural Organization, Social Structure and Value in Italy: Amoral Familism Reconsidered', *American Anthropologist*, 70(1): 1–20.

Simons R. and C. Hughes. 1985. *The Culture-bound Psychiatric Syndromes: Folk Illnesses of Psychiatric and Anthropological Interest*. Reidel: Dordrecht.

Sklar, D. 2001. *Dancing with the Virgin: Body and Faith in the Fiesta of Tortugas, New Mexico*. Berkeley: University of California Press.

Spencer, P. 1985. *Society and the Dance: the Social Anthropology of Process and Performance*. Cambridge: Cambridge University Press.

Sperber, D. 1996. 'Why are Perfect Animals, Hybrids and Monsters Food for Symbolic Thought?' *Method and Theory in the Study of Religion*, 8(2): 143–69.

Stanislavski, K. 1980a. *An Actor Prepares*. London, Methuen.

––––––. 1980b. *Building a Character*. London, Methuen.

––––––. 1981. *Creating a Rôle*. London, Methuen.

Stifani, L. 2000. *Io al santo ci credo. Diario di un musico delle tarantate*. Lecce: Aramirè.

Stokes, M. (ed.). 1994. *Ethnicity, Identity and Music: the Musical Construction of Place*. Oxford: Berg.

Stoller, P. 1989. *The Taste of Ethnographic Things*. Philadelphia: University of Pennsylvania Press.

Storace, S. 1753. 'A Genuine Letter from an Italian Gentleman Concerning the Bite of the Tarantula', *Gentleman's Magazine*, XXIII: 433–34.

Swinburne, H. 1783. *Travels in the Two Sicilies*. London: Elmsely.

Tak, H. 2000. *South Italian Festivals: A Local History of Ritual and Change*. Amsterdam: Amsterdam University Press.

Tamblé, M. 2000. 'Tarantismo e stregoneria. Un legame possibile', in G. Di Mitri (ed.), *Quarant'anni dopo De Martino*. Nardò: Besa, pp. 101–7.

Tarantino, L. 2001. *La notte dei tamburi e dei coltelli. La danza-scherma nel Salento*. Nardò: Besa.

Taylor, J. 1998. *Paper Tangos*. Durham: Duke University Press.

Tentori, T. 1976. 'Social Classes and Family in a Southern Italian Town: Matera', in J. Peristiany (ed.). *Mediterranean Family Structures*. Cambridge: Cambridge University Press, pp. 273–85.

Thayer, L. 2005. 'Tarantismo and Neotarantismo: The Transformation of Ritual in the Wake of Globalization in Southern Italy', in O. Pi-Sunyer (ed.), *The Organization of Diversity: Essays on a Changing Europe*. Research Reports Number 31. Amhurst: University of Massachusetts, pp. 261–90.

Thomas, H. 2003. *The Body, Dance, and Cultural Theory*. Basingstoke: Palgrave MacMillan.

Thorndike, L. 1934. *A History of Magic and Experimental Science*, Vol. 3. New York: Columbia University Press, pp. 526–34.

Tolledi, F. 1998. *Tamburi e coltelli*. Taviano: Quaderni di Astragali.

Tomlinson, G. 1994. *Music in Renaissance Magic: Toward a Historiography of Others*. Chicago: University of Chicago Press.

Torgovnick, M. 1996. *Primitive Passions: Men, Women and the Quest for Ecstasy*. Chicago: Chicago University Press.

Torsello, S. 1997a. 'Alessano: la leggenda di San Paolo', in L. Chiriatti (ed.), *Tarantismo*. Tricase: Arti Grafiche Laborgraf, pp. 60–70.

———. 1997b. 'L'Incubatio: santi, sogni e guarigioni', *Pietre. Speciale feste*, 5: 5.

———. 2007. 'La Notte della taranta. Dall'Istituto Diego Carpitella alla Fondazione La Notte della taranta,' *Idomeneo, Rivista della società di storia patria per la Puglia*, Sezione di Lecce, 9: 15–33.

Trono, C. 2005. 'La cappella di San Paolo fra i luoghi del cuore FAI,' retrieved on 19 March 2006 from www.pizzicata.it.

Tullio-Altan, C. 1976. *Valori, classi sociali, scelte politiche: indagine sulla gioventú degli anni settanta*. Milan: Bompiani.

Turchini, A. 1987. *Morso, morbo, morte: la tarantola fra cultura medica e terapia popolare*. Milan: Franco Angeli.

Turnbull, A. 1771. 'Concerning Italy, the Alledged Effects of the Bite of the Tarantula, and Grecian Antiquities', in *Essays and Observations of the Philosophical Society*. Edinburgh: John Balfour, pp. 100–9.

Turner, B. 1992. *Regulating Bodies*. London: Routledge.

Turner, V. 1982. *From Ritual to Theatre: the Human Seriousness of Play*. New York: Performing Arts Journals.

———. 1989. *The Anthropology of Performance*. Cambridge, MA: Performing Arts Journals.

Urry, J. 2000. *Sociology Beyond Societies*. London: Routledge.

Valetta, L. 1706. *De phalangio apulo*. Naples: Ex tipographia de Bonis.

Vallone, G. 2004. *Le donne guaritrici nella terra del rimorso*. Galatina: Congedo.

Vandenbroeck, P. 1997. *Vols d'âmes: traditions de transe afro-européennes*. Ghent: Snoeck-Ducaju and Zoon.

Vendola, N. 2005. 'Vendola: la mia Taranta,' *La Repubblica*, 27 August: IX.

Wagner, R. 1986. *Symbols that Stand for Themselves*. Chicago: Chicago University Press.

Walpole, H. [1764] 2006. *The Castle of Otranto: A Story*, trans. W. Marshall. Fairfield: First World Library.

Walter, D. 2000. 'The Medium of the Message: Shamanism as Localised Practice in the Nepal Himalayas', in N. Price (ed.), *The Archaeology of Shamanism*, London: Routledge, pp. 105–19.

Washabaugh, W. 1996. *Flamenco: Passion, Politics and Popular Culture*. Oxford: Berg.

Williams, D. [1991] 2004. *Anthropology and the Dance: Ten Lectures*, 2nd edn. Urbana: University of Illinois Press.

You, H. 1994. 'Defining Rhythm: Aspects of an Anthropology of Rhythm'. *Culture, Medicine and Psychiatry*, 18: 361–84.

Young, A. 1982. 'The Anthropologies of Illness and Sickness', *Annual Review of Anthropology*, 11: 257–85.

Zanetti, Z. 1978. *La medicina delle nostre donne*. Foligno: Ediclio.

Zarrilli, P. 2000. *When the Body Becomes All Eyes: Paradigms, Discourses and Practices of Power in Kalarippayattu, a South Indian Martial Art*. Oxford: Oxford University Press.

Filmography

Alla Bua. 2003. *I video 2002–2003*. Ethnosphere.

Bevilacqua, F. 1995. *Stretti nello spazio senza tempo: viaggio nel tarantismo salentino*.

Canizzaro, P. 2001/2003 *La notte della taranta e dintorni*.

———. 2003. *Ritorno a Kurumuny*.

———. 2005. *Ritratti dal Salento*.

Capani, G. 2004. *Un ritmo per l'anima: tarantismo e terapie naturali*.

Carpitella, D. 1960. *La terapia coreutico-musicale del tarantismo*

Ciuffitelli, M. 2005b. *Pizzica with a New York Accent*.

Colopi, A. and C. Giagnotti. 2008. *Mascarimirì. 10 anni, la storia*.

Daudy, M. 2001. *Pizziche de Core*.

Durante, R. 1989. *La Sposa di San Paolo*.

Fersini, M. 2005. *Santu Roccu. La pizzica scherma*.

Gallone, A. 2006. *Amavete!*

Marengo, D. 2005. *Craj – Domani*.

Mingozzi, G. 1982. *Sulla terra del rimorso*.

Miscuglio, A., M. Belmonti and R. Daopoulo. 1981. *Morso d'amore: viaggio attraverso il tarantismo pugliese*.

Pisanelli, P. 2005. *Il sibilo lungo della taranta: musiche e poesie sui percorsi del ragno del Salento*.

Santoro, L. and R. Durante. 1993. *Viaggio a Galatina*.

Stegmueller, R. and R. Koeplin. 1992. *Der Tanz der kleinen Spinne: Tarantella*.

Winspeare, E. 1989. *San Paolo e la tarantola*.

———. 1994. *La Pizzicata*.

———. 2000. *Sangue Vivo*.

Index